Integrated Dental Treatment Planning

Integrated Dental Treatment Planning

a case-based approach

Elizabeth J. Kay
Professor of Dental Health Services Research
Turner Dental School
Manchester, UK

Ann C. Shearer
Consultant in Restorative Dentistry
Dundee Dental School
Dundee, UK

Andrew M. Bridgman
Honorary Lecturer in Law and Ethics for Dentistry
Turner Dental School
Manchester, UK

Gerald M. Humphris
Chair of Health Psychology
Bute Medical School
University of St Andrews
St Andrews, UK

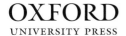

OXFORD
UNIVERSITY PRESS

OXFORD

UNIVERSITY PRESS

Great Clarendon Street, Oxford OX2 6DP

Oxford University Press is a department of the University of Oxford.
It furthers the University's objective of excellence in research, scholarship,
and education by publishing worldwide in

Oxford   New York
Auckland   Cape Town   Dar es Salaam   Hong Kong   Karachi
Kuala Lumpur   Madrid   Melbourne   Mexico City   Nairobi
New Delhi   Shanghai   Taipei   Toronto

With offices in
Argentina   Austria   Brazil   Chile   Czech Republic   France   Greece
Guatemala   Hungary   Italy   Japan   South Korea   Poland   Portugal
Singapore   Switzerland   Thailand   Turkey   Ukraine   Vietnam

Oxford is a registered trade mark of Oxford University Press
in the UK and in certain other countries

Published in the United States
by Oxford University Press Inc., New York

A catalogue record for this title is available from the British Library

Library of Congress Cataloging in Publication Data attached

Integrated dental treatment planning: a case-based approach /
Elizabeth J. Kay [et al.].

Includes index.
1. Dentistry – case studies.   2. Dentist and patient. [DNLM: 1. Dental Care – Case Reports:
2. Dentist–Patient Relations. 3. Patient Care Planning – Case Reports.   WU 29 I605 2005]
RK51.5.I55   2005   617.6′09–dc22   2004 019167

ISBN 0 19 852889 2 (Pbk: alk. paper)

10 9 8 7 6 5 4 3 2 1

Typeset by EXPO Holdings Sdn Bhd., Malaysia.

Printed in Great Britain
on acid-free paper by Ashford Colour Press Ltd., Gosport, Hants

How to use this book

This book is about people, rather than dentistry. So often we compartmentalize 'dentistry' into a category which separates it from 'people' and yet, ultimately, dentistry is about making people healthy. Mouths cannot be ill, upset, sad, or illegal—but problems relating to their mouths can make people ill, upset, sad, or illegal! So this book is about people. It does not purport to teach dentistry, but instead tries to show how dental health and the dental care people receive can profoundly affect their well-being. The book is written for health-care professionals, which is what all members of the dental team are. In each chapter of this book is a 'case story'. In each story, the dental life of a person over several years is described. First, the story is simply told and discussion points and questions are raised. The idea is that you will think through any questions the story raises in your mind and your views on how the patient should be treated. You may also wish to look up any aspects of the clinical, psychological, social, legal or ethical issues in the story which you are unsure of. The purpose of the simplified story is so that you can read it, seek any background information you lack, but most of all so that you can then discuss the case with both your peers and your tutors.

Next, in each chapter the story is repeated, but comments on the case from a barrister, a restorative consultant, a psychologist, and a dentist are added. These are not meant to imply that these are the only aspects of the case worth discussing, they are simply there to offer various insights into different aspects of the case.

Most importantly, the authors would welcome readers' thoughts and feedback. It may be that you disagree with the actions of the dentists in the stories. Indeed, we hope that this *is* the case. But please let us know how you would have acted, what you would have done, or what you think is the 'right' treatment for those patients described. Or, you may feel that there are crucial aspects of the cases which we have overlooked. If so, we do implore you to let us know. Your comments will be collated and hopefully incorporated into future editions of the book, thus making it richer, and almost, we hope, 'interactive'. Your contributions, either from groups or individuals, will be acknowledged. We can be contacted at:

University Dental Hospital of Manchester
Higher Cambridge Street
Manchester M15 6FH, UK

We very much hope you enjoy the book and that it will be used in the spirit in which it was intended—that is, as a platform for discussion, with experts in various fields offering their 'takes' on the cases. The book was never intended as a textbook, or a 'how-to' book. It is here to stimulate thoughts about the wider issues involved in looking after people—which is (although perhaps we sometimes forget this) what dentists and their teams do.

E.J.K.

Foreword

We now accept that lifelong learning should be the quest for every health care professional whether student, graduate, or established practitioner. However, now there are additional learning requirements: mandatory continuing professional development and on the horizon for the dentist, revalidation. In this changing scene for all members of the dental team there is the overwhelming need for exciting educational initiatives to ensure learning is relevant, informative, and fun.

Therefore, I was pleased to be invited to write the foreword for a new style of book embracing an interactive approach. Professor Kay and her collaborating authors are to be congratulated on providing us with an intellectual yet stimulating dental adventure about real people.

Refreshingly, in this book the case history is the framework for the learning process and it is not, as frequently happens, added as an afterthought as a footnote or, worse still, relegated to the appendix. My initial reaction to the briefest of contents pages that I have ever seen, was to wonder how sufficient information could be transmitted through the six chosen patient stories. My doubts were quickly dispelled when I embarked on reading first the simple version of the dental life experiences of the person, which was recounted over a period of time and for some patients this meant as long as ten or twenty years. But more excitement was in store, because after the introduction the stories were fleshed out in depth. The social as well as clinical histories were explored along with associated issues which meant tapping into legal, specialist, and medical expertise.

At the end of reading each of the six case stories I felt truly acquainted with each person, their family, and their problems as well as the solutions. It is rare for a reader to take part in a dental journey of the patient, since we suffer in our profession, as in many others, from the 'little box syndrome' which has so thwarted the art of discovery and the realization of the benefits of an holistic approach for our patients.

Unusually, the authors state that their aim was to provoke, to disagree, and for us to be moved 'to hurl the book across the room'. Cleverly this physical act is tempered by the encouragement to engage in debate and discussion. It is especially commendable that the authors, having successfully stirred such emotions, show maturity and courage to provide contact details so that meaningful exchanges with them can take place with the intention that succeeding editions will benefit from this feedback.

Integrated dental treatment planning is a book that simply cannot be ignored. It encourages in a unique way a partnership in learning which will result in improved patient care; the goal for every health care professional. I will certainly rise to the challenge and send my comments to the authors. I am also confident that after you have read this book you will be doing the same, thus ensuring a truly enjoyable interactive learning experience.

Dame Margaret Seward
Former Chief Dental Officer (England)
Former President of the General Dental Council

Preface

All of the case histories (or case stories as we prefer to call them) in this book are based on real treatment planning dilemmas and loosely based on the characteristics of real patients or amalgams of real patients with whom the authors have played a dental professional role. The authors make no claims that the treatment choices described in this book were the 'right' ones.

Each case attempts to describe the dental, psychological, social, legal, and ethical issues influencing treatment planning. It is hoped that the reader will ponder on the treatment options presented for each case at various stages in each of the 'case stories'. Perhaps the reader would have made different, perhaps better decisions, leading to different outcomes for the patient. The point of the book is that the best restorative treatment planning can go horribly wrong, or surprisingly well, depending on the context of the patient's life and the dentist's professional understanding, knowledge, and skill. It is the authors' hope that readers will contemplate how they might have done things differently, how they might have altered the dentally related events in the lives of the subjects of the case stories and where and how even slight differences in the way patients were dealt with might have had a huge impact.

The point of writing these 'longitudinal' cases is to try to enhance readers' awareness that the sequelae of their own actions depend not only on dental pathologies but also on how the patient is judged, how the dentist relates to the patient, and how the dentist can best meet his or her duty of care in difficult circumstances. Only by examining the outcomes of our professional decisions in the long term, in years and decades, rather than weeks or months, can we begin to fully understand our professional roles and responsibilities.

We hope that you find the case stories interesting and intriguing. Indeed, we hope that sometimes you might want to hurl the book across the room, shouting: 'But that was stupid, you *shouldn't* have done that'. So long as you can answer the question 'why not' when you disagree with what was done in the case stories, then the book will have served its purpose!

E.J.K.

Acknowledgements

We would first like to thank all the patients and people upon whom the 'case stories' in this book are loosely based. We hope they will not take offence at any poetic licence we may have taken whilst writing about them.

Secondly, we owe great gratitude to Dr Iain Mackie and Dr Liz Turbill, both of whom provided us with photographic material.

Lastly, and most importantly, we would like to thank Miss Pam Brown who has collated and typed the manuscripts. This has been a very complex book to coordinate and the work involved in amalgamating four people's writings has been immense. We are deeply grateful to Pam, without whom there would be no book!

Contents

1 Tilly: a Lancashire mill worker

Tilly is aged 63. She presents complaining that her full upper denture 'looks horrible' and is 'coming loose'.

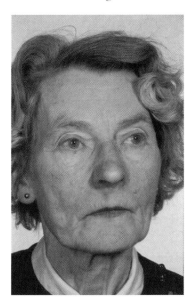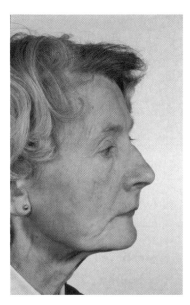

Tilly, aged 63 years

By questioning Tilly, the dentist discovers that Tilly's husband died the previous year of cancer so she now lives on her own in a socially deprived Lancashire mill town. She has not attended the dentist since her upper teeth were extracted for her wedding when she was 21.

Why would someone have their teeth extracted for their wedding?

Tilly has two daughters, one of whom lives 10 miles from her but whom she rarely sees. Her other daughter does not visit, as the son-in-law did not see 'eye to eye' with Tilly's late husband when he was alive. Her only son lives abroad but visits at Christmas.

What is the dental significance of Tilly's social history?

As a person, Tilly seems rather anxious and jumpy although she claims not to be nervous about dentistry. She repeatedly states that she does not wish to be any trouble and that she will probably manage with her dentures if the dentist can just 'adjust' them.

How could the dentist check Tilly's emotional responses to visiting the dentist?

Tilly states that she cleans her teeth every day. On examination, the dentist finds that Tilly has a very poorly fitting upper denture, the acrylic of which is bleached as white as the teeth.

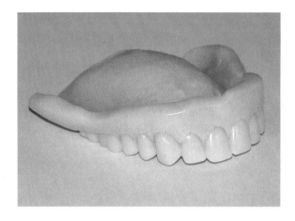

Tilly's upper denture

How could the pink acrylic of a denture have become so white?

Tilly's occlusal relationship appears to be Class III but it is difficult to get her to bite in a retruded contact. Tilly tells the dentist that she has not eaten in front of anyone other than her husband for the past 20 years, not even, she confides, at her daughter's wedding reception.

What impact have Tilly's dentures had on her day-to-day life?

The mucosa beneath Tilly's denture is inflamed, with an appearance of chronic (atrophic) candidiasis. On palpation of the upper ridge, you think you can feel an unerupted posterior tooth. Radiographs confirm the presence of an

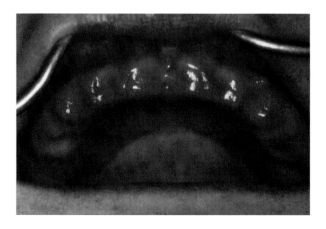

An example of denture stomatitis

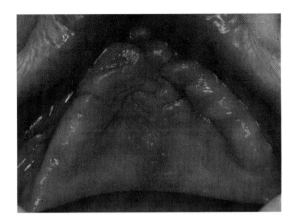

An example of a flabby ridge

unerupted UR8. There is also a large ulcer on the tip of Tilly's tongue. The upper anterior ridge is mobile and 'flabby' and when Tilly speaks, the upper denture has a noticeable tendency to drop.

What is causing Tilly's dentures to be so unstable?

In the lower jaw, Tilly has incisors, canines, and first premolars. She says that LL1 broke about 2 weeks ago when she was eating a toffee. She says that it is not painful now, nor was it when it broke. When you question Tilly further about the ulcer on her tongue, she admits that the gap in her teeth has made her tongue sore and that, although she doesn't mind the space looking a bit 'funny', she says that it does affect her speech.

All of the remaining lower teeth have abrasion cavities and LR4 and LL4 are carious, both cervically and occlusally.

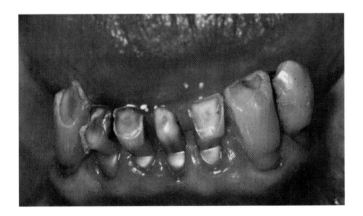

Lower anterior teeth with abrasion cavities

What are Tilly's immediate and more long-term problems and how would you treat them?

How would you check that the ulcer was not sinister?

Tilly reports that she is fit and well, and although attending the surgery is difficult and takes an hour on the bus, she is happy to have whatever treatment the dentist deems to be best.

Tilly says that she has never had, or worn, a lower denture and that she does not think she would cope with one.

The dentist decides to provide a new upper denture and an overdenture on the lower canine teeth and proceeds to extract the lower teeth other than LR 3 and LL 3 and then provides Tilly with a lower overdenture abutting on these teeth.

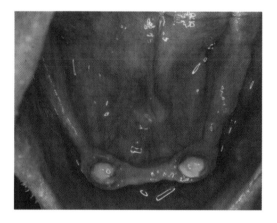

Lower canines as abutments for a complete lower denture

What factors must be taken into consideration when planning an overdenture?

Three years later: Tilly presents again in the autumn. She says she has lost her lower denture and would like a new one.

On examination, there is gingival overgrowth on the overdenture abutments and little evidence that the original lower overdenture has been worn, but Tilly has kept the abutments clean and they seem sound.

On questioning, Tilly states that the lower denture was fine 'just a bit of a mouthful' and that she has lost it and that she cannot imagine what could have become of it. She wonders whether, while you do the lower you might also do the upper, so that she can have smaller, whiter teeth.

Should the dentist provide a new denture?

Should the dentist provide treatment to fit with the patient's wishes?

Tilly is now reunited with her estranged daughter (who has divorced her husband) and is looking forward to a family reunion at Christmas, when she will meet her first grandchild (her son's son) for the first time. A christening is planned and Tilly seems excited and a little anxious about the preparations.

On checking the medical history, Tilly tells the dentist that the doctor has given her some tablets 'for her nerves'. She does not have them with her, nor can she remember what they are called.

Can the dentist proceed with treatment without knowing what these tablets are?

The dentist agrees to make Tilly a new upper full denture and lower overdenture.

During the visits while the new dentures are being made, Tilly talks a great deal about her family and the impending reunion. Tilly tells you that she will bring some pictures of the party.

Should the dentist encourage Tilly's friendship?

The dentist and Tilly engage in some debate about the size and shade of the teeth on the new dentures.

How should you decide on the best tooth-shade for a patient?

Tilly wants A1, while the dentist is convinced that, given her age, the shape of her face and her skin tones, that C2 would give a far more pleasing end result. In the end they agree to compromise on B1.

When the dentures are delivered Tilly is thrilled with her new appearance.

After this, each year in autumn, Tilly reappears. Each year the dentures have either been lost, or broken, or she says they have 'rubbed her gum'. Usually Tilly brings with her a bag full of problem dentures so that she can show the dentist the problems and point out which teeth she liked best in terms of appearance.

Seven years or so pass, with Tilly making annual requests. You notice that she is becoming more and more demanding in her requests. You also notice that her appearance is not as smart as it used to be. She seems not to be looking after herself as she used to.

Your options in the face of Tilly's increasing demands are:

1.   To do nothing and send her away as her 'dental' need is limited.
2.   Continue to make her what she requests even though it is uncertain whether it is in her best dental interests, because she benefits from the visits in other ways.

Is it the dentist's duty to help patients in non-clinical ways?

3.   Organize some sort of social care for Tilly so that she becomes less dependent on support and company from the dental surgery.

Is organization of social support within a dentist's duty of care?

Ten years later: The same dentist receives a telephone call from a local residential home for the elderly, requesting that he visit one of the old ladies who lives at the home.

How can dentistry be provided at people's homes?

He duly attends the residence where, on arrival, the matron of the home says that they have a lady suffering from severe senile dementia who appears to be in considerable pain. The matron thinks the pain is emanating from the lady's mouth. Matron informs you that the patient is an insulin-dependent diabetic.

What is senile dementia and how will it affect Tilly's dental treatment?
Is insulin-dependent diabetes relevant to Tilly's dental treatment?

It is agreed that the dentist will do his best to solve any dental problems and he asks the lady's name. He is told it is Tilly. He enquires as to whether the lady used to attend his surgery but the matron is unsure.

On meeting the patient, the dentist sees at once it is indeed the same Tilly although unsurprisingly there is no glimmer of recognition from her. It is not possible to take a history as Tilly only stares dumbly when questions are asked.

There seems to be a slight swelling of the right side of Tilly's face. However, when the dentist tries to examine her, Tilly shrinks away and becomes extremely distressed when the dentist continues to attempt the examination. She is in danger of injuring both herself or one of the members of staff. As she yells, the dentist sees that the over-denture abutments are still present but clearly no oral hygiene measures have been undertaken for some time.

Should the dentist insist on examining Tilly, when she does not wish to be examined?

You discuss the matter with the matron who tells you that Tilly is sometimes rather aggressive and almost always demanding. She has no known medical problems, other than her diabetes, and she is incontinent because of her Alzheimer's. Matron says there is one daughter who visits occasionally but she is not aware of any other living relatives. Matron is also aware that Tilly has been a widow for many years.

All the staff at the home have noticed Tilly clutching at the right side of her face in increasing desperation, sometimes in tears. Unfortunately, Tilly's communicative powers are so diminished that she is unable to tell anyone what her problem is, although sometimes the desperation in her eyes is all too obvious.

Diagnosis

Tilly appears to have a swelling, very probably of dental origin. On consulting Tilly's previous notes the dentist becomes aware that a buried UR8 may well be the cause of the problem. However, diagnosis without examination is problematic.

Treatment options

1. Do nothing.
2. Forcibly examine the patient, perhaps under sedation, with a view to treating any problems, if appropriate, with antibiotics and pain killers.
3. Organize examination under general anaesthetic, plus extraction of UR8.

Which of these treatment options is in Tilly's best interest?

TILLY: A LANCASHIRE MILL WORKER

Tilly is aged 63. She presents complaining that her full upper denture 'looks horrible' and is 'coming loose'.

By questioning Tilly, the dentist discovers that her husband died the previous year of cancer so she now lives on her own in a socially deprived Lancashire mill town. She has not attended the dentist since her upper teeth were extracted for her wedding when she was 21.

At the beginning of the twentieth century the eminent physician William Hunter blamed oral sepsis for 'chronic dyspepsias, intestinal disorders, ill health, anaemias and nervous complaints'. The term oral sepsis was later changed to 'focal infection' and this condition was blamed for many systemic diseases. What followed in dentistry was the avoidance of operative dentistry in favour of extractions. Any teeth that were endodontically or periodontally involved (whether symptomatic or asymptomatic) were extracted to avoid a possible focus for infection. This situation prevailed for the first half of the twentieth century until the theory of focal infection started to fall out of favour. This meant that up until the 1950s many people had teeth extracted that would not be extracted today. The extractions often involved complete arches of teeth, especially if there was any periodontal disease (or 'pyorrhoea'). Extractions and the provision of dentures were frequently carried out in young people and consequently many elderly people now consider dentistry to be unpleasant and painful. In the north of England and Scotland, girls customarily had all their teeth extracted and dentures constructed prior to marriage as part of their trousseau.

The consequences of early tooth loss are seen now in our elderly edentulous population. They have marked loss of alveolar bone and some loss of muscle tone and as a result they find denture wearing very difficult. The dentures may have poor stability and retention and this can result in loss of enjoyment in eating and other social embarrassment.

Tilly has two daughters, one of whom lives 10 miles from her but whom she rarely sees. Her other daughter does not visit, as the son in law did not see 'eye to eye' with Tilly's late husband when he was alive. Her only son lives abroad but visits at Christmas.

Many studies have shown that social isolation can have a detrimental effect upon a person's general health. Obviously, social support plays an important role in enhancing health-related behaviours, as well as providing emotional support and enhancing a person's sense of self-worth (in itself important for health). Bereavement changes the availability of social support, especially when a spouse dies. Tilly is likely to undergo a number of lifestyle changes that may have an impact on her health. Not least, she may experience greater financial difficulties with the loss of her husband's income. Elderly women living alone are amongst the most impoverished people in Britain. It is not difficult to imagine how such factors could lead to a general deterioration in her health.

As a person, Tilly seems rather anxious and jumpy although she claims not to be nervous about dentistry. She repeatedly states that she does not wish to be any trouble and that she will probably manage with her dentures if the dentist can just 'adjust' them.

Tilly claimed that she was not unduly nervous about dental treatment. Simply inviting her to complete a standard dental anxiety questionnaire such as Corah's Dental Anxiety Scale or the Modified Dental Anxiety Scale (MDAS) could check this. As mentioned elsewhere in this book the MDAS is preferred because it includes a question about local anaesthesia, has a standard answering system for each of its five questions and is simple to complete, score, and compare with normative data. However, the dentist may sense that dental anxiety is not the main emotional response experienced by Tilly when visiting the dentist. There are a number of other possibilities:

1. She is socially awkward and perhaps even socially phobic and finds it difficult to share personal information with the dentist about her difficulties.
2. She is anxious, but not necessarily about dental treatment. She has an ulcer in her mouth, which she may or may not be aware of. If she is aware of the ulcer then she may be worried that it signifies a possible health problem.
3. She is embarrassed about her dental condition and poor attendance history.

These three possibilities can be assessed through judicious questioning.

The first issue can be broached with the patient by asking how she feels about talking of her dental problems with the dentist. Active listening will encourage the patient to disclose.

The second issue of concern can be raised by asking the patient whether they have noticed the presence of an ulcer in the mouth. If she states that she has not, this would mean that no symptoms or sensations have been noticed by the patient and so there is little likelihood of the patient being unduly anxious about the ulcer. However, the dentist should be mindful that the patient may wish to convey a confident manner in the hope that any concerns about the ulcer can be ignored, a process known as denial. Further questioning will be necessary to exclude this, admittedly minor, possibility.

The third and final issue of embarrassment is of interest as this can be a frequent concern of patients. Dentists should try to identify this difficulty in their patients, as it will enable an active strategy of encouraging disclosure in the patient. If the dentist is successful in encouraging the patient to share their embarrassment about the condition of their teeth/mouth and past poor attendance record then the dentist can reassure by:

- Starting to explain how well she has done to admit that this is a difficulty. Congratulating her in making a positive step in trying to resolve her dental problems.
- Gently invite her to comment on previous experiences with dentists in the past. It is possible that her experience has not been positive with health professionals in the past and she may have suffered from active 'victim blaming'. For example, a common complaint by patients is that clinicians tell them that they should have attended much earlier when far easier and less costly treatments would have been possible. The dentist must try to resist this even though it is likely to be correct—earlier diagnosis and treatment is nearly always simpler and less invasive and is also more likely to be completely successful.
- State that it is the dentist's job to assist the patient to return them to a state of dental 'fitness'.
- Start explaining the possible options for treatment and what the patient can do to assist in ensuring that the treatment can be successful.

A further explanation for Tilly's reticence for receipt of dental treatment may be put forward. She may when young have been subject to sexual, physical or emotional abuse or neglect which is known to be a factor in the development and maintenance of dental fear. A North American survey showed that women with a history of trauma were more likely to show elevated levels of dental fear. The embarrassing and shameful feelings associated with abuse and neglect would not make this an easy area for patients to discuss or admit to and would possibly reduce the likelihood of volunteering information about dental anxiety.

Tilly states that she cleans her teeth every day. On examination, the dentist finds that Tilly has a very poorly fitting upper denture, the acrylic of which is bleached as white as the teeth.

Bleaching of dentures occurs because the dentures are being placed in an immersion cleanser at too high a temperature (>50°C) or for too long.

Patients should be advised to care for their dentures as follows:
- When not being worn dentures should be placed in cold water after being cleaned.
- Dentures should be cleaned every night. This can be done with soap and a nailbrush. A denture brush or toothbrush may be used but not ordinary toothpaste, as this is too abrasive for dentures. Effervescent tablet cleaners are quite efficient, but are more expensive. If a tablet cleaner is used, use it perhaps once a week and do not use water that is more than lukewarm as high temperatures will damage the material of the dentures.
- While cleaning hold the denture over a basin of water or a towel so that breakage is less likely should the denture be dropped.

Tilly's occlusal relationship appears to be Class III, but it is difficult to get her to bite in a retruded contact. Tilly tells the dentist that she has not eaten in front of anyone other than her husband for the past 20 years, not even, she confides, at her daughter's wedding reception.

Here it is possible to see how quite basic dental issues can be a cause of severe social disablement for the individual. Superficially, one might imagine that dental problems are primarily functional. For instance, Tilly's poorly fitting denture seems to have caused basic functional problems in terms of chewing, eating and possibly pain when eating different kinds of food. But it is clear here, as in the case of many dentally related problems, that the implications extend far beyond such functional behaviour and into the interpersonal and social realm. This is perhaps not surprising when one thinks about the way in which human food intake and eating behaviour is very much a social phenomenon. Eating and meal times tend to be associated with other people—they are times when we come together not just to eat but to chat and socialize. Many patients with denture problems find that their basic enjoyment of food diminishes because the physical problems of the denture have an impact on their interactive encounters. For instance, it may take a person longer to finish a meal than others in the group, and so they feel embarrassed as everyone seems to be sitting around waiting and watching. A person may be embarrassed about the noise they are making when chewing food. The 'faulty' appearance of the denture from the point of view of the patient may mean that they avoid laughing or smiling in front of other people, even to the point where they avoid conversation and interaction with others. In this sense, it is clear that denture problems may potentiate quite severe social and interpersonal problems.

It is clearly evident that Tilly's dental problems are having a detrimental effect upon her everyday social functioning. Her speech has also been affected. Similarly to eating behaviour, our language and ability to speak 'normally' is one of the primary ways in which we make contact with others in our world. If a person's ability to speak 'normally' is affected, clearly, this could have a detrimental effect upon basic social interaction. Such people may increasingly begin to dread occasions when they have to socialize and interact with other people. This could, in the worst-case scenario, result in withdrawal, social isolation and a negative spiral in which the individual loses confidence in him/herself and draws further away from the social world.

Although the aesthetic needs of patients may not seem particularly important for clinical treatment *per se*, as is clear, such concerns are of paramount importance from the patient's perspective. For instance, some studies have shown that a person's positive 'aesthetic' sense, and a sense of their own facial attractiveness is positively correlated with higher ratings of self-esteem. Clearly, dental problems can therefore have important psychosocial reverberations.

This can perhaps be most clearly seen when one considers people with dental problems and their association with low self-esteem. For instance, studies of children with clefts have shown that they are at significant risk for social competence problems relating to the development of friendships, progress in school, and participation in organizations. Problems with social competence are likely to have a detrimental effect on development. It has been found that adults with repaired clefts are less likely to marry than their non-cleft siblings and they have more problems with social withdrawal. Dental care obviously has the potential to make a positive contribution to facial attractiveness, and the potential psychosocial reverberations related to facial attractiveness.

However, it is important to stress a note of caution when making generalizations about the links between psychosocial issues and dental problems. For instance, in one study a group of adolescents with mild to moderate malocclusions underwent orthodontic treatment. They were assessed pre- and post-treatment on a battery of psychological and social measures. Post-treatment, although it was found that self-evaluations of dental/facial attractiveness improved significantly, treatment actually failed to have any effect on self-reported self-esteem or social competency. Although important to bear in mind the connection between dental/facial appearance and psychological issues such as self-esteem, it is also important not to over-estimate their effects.

The mucosa beneath Tilly's denture is inflamed, with an appearance of chronic (atrophic) candidiasis. On palpation of the upper ridge, you think you can feel an unerupted posterior tooth. Radiographs confirm the presence of an unerupted UR8. There is also a large ulcer on the tip of Tilly's tongue. The upper anterior ridge is mobile and 'flabby' and when Tilly speaks, the upper denture has a noticeable tendency to drop.

The stability of dentures is a balance between the retaining forces and the displacing forces. Tilly's ability to control her dentures is influenced by this balance. The following are likely causes for the instability of Tilly's dentures:
- Decreased retaining forces:
    - lack of peripheral seal,
    - inelasticity of cheek tissues,
    - dry mouth,
    - poor neuromuscular control,
    - air between fitting surface and tissues caused by ridge resorption.
- Increased displacing forces:
    - poor fit to supporting tissues,
    - denture not in optimal space,
    - occlusal errors,
    - fibrous displaceable 'flabby' ridge,
    - pain avoidance mechanisms.

In the lower jaw, Tilly has incisors, canines, and first premolars. She says that LL1 broke about 2 weeks ago when she was eating a toffee. She says that it is not painful now, nor was it when it broke. When you question Tilly further about the ulcer on her tongue, she admits that the gap in her teeth has made her tongue sore and that, although she doesn't mind the space looking a bit 'funny', she says that it does affect her speech.

All of the remaining lower teeth have abrasion cavities and LR4 and LL4 are carious, both cervically and occlusally.

TILLY'S FIRST VISIT

Immediate problems on Tilly's first visit:
- She has not had dental treatment for 32 years.
- She has an ulcer on her tongue.
- Fractured tooth LL1.
- Candidiasis.

Tongue ulcer

The most likely cause for this is the fractured tooth, and this should certainly be dealt with first. The possibility of the ulcer being malignant is unlikely but the patient can questioned on possible risk factors. The tooth should be dressed, if no decision has been made about whether to retain it, or it should be restored or extracted.

Fractured tooth

This is an aesthetic problem as well as the probable cause of Tilly's ulcer. It does not, however, appear to be causing her any pain. This may be because the fracture is small or because the pulp is non-vital or the root canal is obliterated by reparative dentine. Beware of the latter as this may preclude root canal treatment.

Candidiasis

This affects between a quarter and two-thirds of denture wearers and is more common in females. It has several causative factors:
- Trauma from dentures.
- Presence of *Candida albicans* or other *Candida* species.
- Systemic factors.

It should be treated before any new denture is made because the tissues will be swollen. If impressions are taken without resolving the candidiasis, the swelling will be duplicated in the new denture. Inflammation then resolves under the new denture resulting in lack of fit and a causative factor is re-established.

Treatment

1. Reduce denture trauma:
   - Add tissue conditioner to the fitting surface to improve fit. Tissue conditioner should be in place for 1 or 2 weeks at most before impressions are recorded for a new denture.
   - Add cold-cure acrylic to the occlusal surface to re-establish occlusion. Correct any other defects in the old dentures, such as freeway space
2. Leave denture out at night: patients should be discouraged from wearing their dentures day and night, although many find this socially unacceptable.
3. Denture hygiene:
   - Brush dentures to remove plaque.
   - Disinfectant—soak overnight in a dilute solution of hypochlorite or chlorhexidine.
4. Antifungal agents: topical amphotericin, nystatin or miconazole should be considered if local measures do not bring about resolution.

If none of these measures resolve the candidiasis, consider the possibilty of an underlying systemic problem and refer to a GP.

Tilly's other dental problems

- Unstable, unretentive, worn and bleached F/– with poor occlusion.
- Only lower anterior teeth present.

The upper denture

- Flabby ridge: This is classically seen under a complete upper denture opposed by lower anterior teeth. The unbalanced occlusion results in resorption of the alveolar bone, which is then replaced by fibrous tissue. Stability of the denture is compromised as a result of the fibrous tissue. For flabby ridges you need to use an impression technique that will not displace the tissues. If the fibrous tissue is distorted, the new denture will fit only when seated by occlusal pressure. When the teeth are apart, elastic recoil of the displaced tissue forces the denture downwards. The new denture should be made on a model cast from an impression of the flabby ridge in its resting position. Your impression technique should involve a material of low viscosity and a spaced tray, possibly perforated as well.
- Poor occlusion: Tilly has worn her upper denture for 32 years. The acrylic has become worn and this has resulted in a loss of occlusal face height. She has adopted a forward posture of her mandible to achieve occlusion between her natural lower teeth and the worn upper denture. It may be possible to correct this using cold-cure acrylic but this is unlikely to give a denture of good appearance.
- Bleached appearance: This is normally caused by use of denture cleaning tablets in water of too high temperature.

Lower arch

The remaining teeth are contributing to the problem of the upper flabby ridge, and because of this it may be argued that they should be extracted. However, Tilly has had no lower posterior teeth for many years and this results in the tongue spreading out and the buccinator muscle attachments moving inwards. This reduces the neutral zone (the area between tongue and cheeks where soft tissue forces acting on a denture are least) and will be one factor in the decision about management of the lower arch and the design of any lower prosthesis.

The unerupted third molar will only have been discovered if a panoramic radiograph has been taken. There does not appear to be any clinical indication for taking such a radiograph. The radiographs of choice in this case are peri-apicals of the lower anteriors. The panoramic is not a helpful view for lower incisors because the shadow of the cervical vertebrae obscures the incisors. There would appear to be no indication for removal of the third molar (see NICE/SIGN guidelines).

Treatment options

1. Do nothing. This is not an option because Tilly has presented with an ulcer. It is highly unlikely that it is malignant, but this possibility must be excluded.
2. Reline/adjust upper denture. It is certainly possible to reline the denture and adjust the occlusal surfaces by adding cold-cure acrylic. This will not result in a very attractive denture but should be considered as a short-term option to allow Tilly to adapt to the changes and to reduce the soft tissue inflammation.
3. Provide new upper/leave lower. This is an attractive option as it is unlikely that Tilly will tolerate a lower denture. A duplicate denture technique (copy denture) would be indicated here because:
   - Tilly has accommodated to the shape of this denture for 32 years.
   - None of Tilly's symptoms are attributable to errors in the polished surfaces.
   - There is wear of the occlusal surfaces.
   - The denture base material and teeth have deteriorated.
4. Provide new upper and lower partial. If the prognosis for the remaining teeth is poor then providing a lower partial denture may allow Tilly to adapt to wearing a lower denture before it is forced on her by the loss of her remaining teeth. A lower partial would give stability to the upper, reduce the trauma to the anterior ridge and give Tilly an opportunity to try a lower partial denture. She will find this difficult because of the tongue spread that will have occurred. Many lower partial dentures are not worn. The main reasons for wearing lower partials is appearance and this may not be a

problem for Tilly. A lower partial denture will increase plaque accumulation and caries rate.

5. Provide a new upper and lower partial with precision attachments. It would be unwise to embark on complex care for a patient who has not had dental treatment for 32 years and who you do not know. It may not offer any real benefits to the patient and aftercare will be needed, which we do not know whether Tilly will comply with.

6. Provide new upper and distal extension resin bonded cantilever bridges. This is an attractive option as it allows for improved stability of the upper denture; however, it carries the same proviso as option 5 regarding complex treatment on a new patient. You would also have to be sure that the remaining lower teeth had a reasonable prognosis.

7. Provide a new upper and overdenture on LL3 and LR3. This is a good option if you have decided that the prognosis of the lower incisors and premolars is very poor. It offers all the advantages of overdentures, namely proprioception/discriminatory ability, alveolar ridge preservation, support, stability, retention, and reduced load on soft tissues and it can be used as a transition to a full lower denture. The disadvantages of this option are the need to carry out two root canal treatments (success rate in cross-sectional studies of 60–70%) and the high caries rate associated with overdenture abutments.

8. Provide full upper and full lower. This is to be avoided unless lower anteriors are unrestorable as Tilly may not be able to accommodate to wearing a lower denture.

Embark on detailed questioning to ascertain the duration of the ulcer's occurrence, severity and painfulness. Also check medical history to obtain any evidence of risk factors, including tobacco smoking and excessive alcohol consumption. Ask the patient what they think the ulcer was caused by, and if they had considered it would need investigating. The patient may be oblivious to the association between painful, non-healing ulcers and malignancy. The public's knowledge of oral cancer is not extensive, due to the rarity of the disease. A balance needs to be struck between not unduly frightening the patient and giving sufficient information so that the patient can understand the need for an investigation. If the ulcer shows features which require further specialist opinion then the patient should be informed that the ulcer needs looking at by a specialist at the local hospital. Both the oral medicine unit and the patient's general medical practitioner need to be contacted. Close attention to the words employed during these conversations between patient and dentist is essential. Too much reassurance that all will be well may be demotivating and the patient may not bother to attend for their diagnostic appointment. However, if there is no discussion of the low probability of significant disease, the patient may jump to conclusions and become extremely anxious.

Tilly reports that she is fit and well, and although attending the surgery is difficult and takes an hour on the bus she is happy to have whatever treatment the dentist deems to be best.

Tilly says that she has never had, or worn, a lower denture and that she does not think she would cope with one.

The dentist decides to provide a new upper denture and an overdenture on the lower canine teeth and proceeds to extract the lower teeth other than LR 3 and LL 3 and then provides Tilly with a lower overdenture abutting on these teeth.

Overdenture abutment teeth are at risk of caries, periodontal disease, and inflammation of any pulpal remnants. Prevalence figures for caries in overdenture abutments range from 15 to 35%. Gingival bleeding is almost universal around overdenture abutments.

Overdentures are not suitable for patients with poor plaque control or with a diet high in refined carbohydrates. Patients who are suitable initially may become unsuitable with increasing disability and loss of manual dexterity. Diets high in refined carbohydrates are common in care homes.

Care of overdenture abutments involves:
- plaque control of teeth,
- plaque control of denture,
- dietary advice,
- topical fluoride treatment,
- maintenance of abutments and dentures.

THREE YEARS LATER

Three years later: Tilly presents again in the autumn. She says she has lost her lower denture and would like a new one.

On examination, there is gingival overgrowth on the overdenture abutments and little evidence that the original lower overdenture has been worn, but Tilly has kept the abutments clean and they seem sound.

On questioning, Tilly states that the lower denture was fine 'just a bit of a mouthful' and that she has lost it and that she cannot imagine what could have become of it. She wonders whether, while you do the lower you might also do the upper, so that she can have smaller, whiter teeth.

The upper denture is just 3 years old. There appears to be no clinical reason to replace it. Tilly's request seems to be purely for cosmetic reasons. In view of Tilly's circumstances it is likely that the denture was provided under the National Health Service Regulations. Tilly may have had to make a contribution towards the cost of her treatment. She may now be completely exempt or may still have to make a contribution. Of course, it is always possible that

Tilly has some small savings and is prepared to pay privately for the new dentures.

If there were sound clinical reasons for replacing Tilly's denture then her request would raise no ethical or legal issues. It is a common request, presumably an attempt to recapture lost youthful appearance. The request for small white teeth is her choice and this can be assumed to be a valid choice as there is no reason to think that Tilly is not fully competent. Similarly, there is no suggestion that a family member or friend is pressurizing Tilly to make the request she has made. Such a request, however, will often run counter to the dentist's desire to recreate a 'natural' dentition. Although in such circumstances a conflict of autonomy arises, given that that no harm is caused by providing small white teeth the decision to do so could not be criticised on ethical grounds. Indeed, it could be argued that psychological/social harm could be caused by the dentist's refusal to do so.

The situation is somewhat different when there are no clinical reasons to replace the denture and the denture is to be provided as NHS treatment, whether or not Tilly makes a full or part contribution. The dentist has a clear and moral duty to protect the NHS budget, which is a limited and finite resource. That resource should not be accessed for treatments without sound clinical justification. There is, as mentioned above, the small risk of harm that may arise from refusal. Whether or not that would present sufficient clinical reason is matter for consideration in the individual circumstance. Tilly has had these dentures for 3 years and the request for dentures is cosmetic and non-therapeutic. The current view is that public funding should not be used to provide for cosmetic 'treatment'.

Crowns and, in particular, veneers are often provided for cosmetic reasons, but the justification for such provision is as follows. Crowns and veneers when used to improve appearance do so by restoring the appearance of teeth to what would be considered to be their normal appearance; the perceived normal in terms of size, shape and colour. Thus, restoration to 'normal' can be considered ethical, even if the treatment is cosmetic, but treatment provided solely to alter the person's appearance, particularly if it makes them look 'less normal' may be unethical. Clear examples of the former are the veneering of teeth with tetracycline and other intrinsic staining, or restoring peg-shaped laterals to a more standard shape. To provide small white teeth, perhaps especially the white, for Tilly is contrary to the expected normal appearance of the teeth of a 63-year-old.

Tilly is now reunited with her estranged daughter (who has divorced her husband) and is looking forward to a family reunion at Christmas, when she will meet her first grandchild (her son's son) for the first time. A christening is planned and Tilly seems excited and a little anxious about the preparations.

On checking the medical history, Tilly tells the dentist that the doctor has given her some tablets 'for her nerves'. She does not have them with her, nor can she remember what they are called.

To provide treatment for a patient without a full and proper medical history is unwise. It can lead to sudden and unexpected problems, with harmful results. Therefore it exposes the patient to a risk of harm and consequently would be regard as unethical. Further, it would be in breach of the General Dental Council's 'Maintaining Standards', which regards the taking of a medical history before commencing treatment as mandatory (Paragraph 4.3 in Maintaining Standards). Finally, were any untoward incident to arise from such failure the dentist may also be found to be negligent. There is no doubt that many courses of dental treatment are undertaken without full knowledge of the patient's medical health or medication. This will usually be when the patient has chosen not to inform the dentist, for whatever reason. There is nothing the dentist can do in such a situation, save to ensure, and be able to show, that a proper and thorough medical history was taken.

Tilly has told the dentist that she is taking tablets for her nerves. She does not know what they are. This in not an emergency situation and there is no need to provide treatment without an opportunity to find out. No doubt Tilly could bring the tablets, or her prescription (as this is likely to be a repeat prescription), with her next time. Failing this, the dentist could ask Tilly's permission to speak to her doctor. There is an argument that in seeking care from health-care professionals the patient gives implied consent to the exchange of information between health-care professionals so long as that exchange is in their best interests. The doctor may not, however, hold to this view. It would probably be correct to seek Tilly's permission before speaking to the doctor.

It is unwise to guess at the drugs a patient is taking, but the possibilities for Tilly are listed below. Fortunately among the drugs listed below there are few interactions with drugs that a dentist could prescribe.

- Anxiolytic drugs such as the benzodiazepines (e.g. diazepam, lorazepam) alleviate anxiety states such as stress-related symptoms, unhappiness, and minor physical disease.
- Beta-blockers (e.g. propranolol) do not affect psychological symptoms such as worry but they do reduce autonomic symptoms such as palpitations or tremor.
- Antipsychotic drugs (e.g. chlorpromazine) are used to quieten disturbed patients such as those with agitated depression. They may also be used for severe anxiety as a short-term measure.
- Antidepressants are effective in the treatment of major depression of moderate and severe degree and for lower-grade chronic depression. The major classes of drugs include the tricyclics (e.g. amitriptyline), the selective serotonin reuptake inhibitors (e.g. fluoxetine) and the monoamine oxidase inhibitors (e.g. phenelzine).

- Monoamine oxidase inhibitors (MAOIs) may be less effective and show dangerous interactions with some foods and drugs. There is no evidence of dangerous interactions between local anaesthetics containing adrenaline (epinephrine) and MAOIs or tricyclic antidepressants. Care should be taken to avoid inadvertent intravenous administration.
- St John's wort is a popular herbal remedy for mild depression; however, it can interact with antidepressants and the two should not be used together.

The dentist agrees to make Tilly a new upper full denture and lower overdenture.

As there is gingival overgrowth this suggests that the surfaces of the overdenture abutment are flat or concave. Such shapes are more likely to collect plaque or be overgrown by the gingivae than convex abutments. If the abutments are to be retained you could either accept the shape or change the shape by replacing the plastic restoration with another more domed plastic restoration or by having gold copings made in the laboratory.

It would be worth trying to find out why Tilly is not wearing her lower denture. If it transpires that she has no intention of ever wearing a lower denture, perhaps because of difficulties in controlling the denture which she describes as ' a bit of a mouthful', then it is a pointless exercise making another denture and changing the abutments. You would be better concentrating on the upper denture which is also causing Tilly some concerns.

If Tilly is determined to try another lower denture then it is important to ensure that it is within the neutral zone and that there is adequate freeway space and correct occlusion.

During the visits while the new dentures are being made., Tilly talks a great deal about her family and the impending reunion. Tilly tells you that she will bring some pictures of the party.

The fact that Tilly feels sufficiently reassured to 'open up' to you as her dentist and discuss her relationships with her family is obviously indicative that a certain amount of trust and rapport has been established. However, it is also important to be cautious of becoming 'over-involved' because, given Tilly's social isolation, this may be a sign that she is becoming increasingly dependent on the interpersonal contact she is receiving during her dental visits. This could encourage dental visiting behaviour less for dental treatment needs and more for basic social interaction. Perhaps suggest to her that she tries to use the occasion of receiving a new denture as the stage for embarking on more social activities.

The dentist and Tilly engage in some debate about the size and shade of the teeth on the new dentures.

Various methods have been proposed for selecting anterior teeth for dentures. The Williams classification suggests matching face shape to tooth shape. There is no evidence for this approach. Another suggestion is to use the personality, sex, and age of the patient to choose the tooth shape. For example, for a delicately featured female the teeth should be slender with rounded incisal edges. In selecting tooth shade, the skin tone can be used as a guide as there is some harmony between skin colour and tooth shade. Age is another guide, as with increasing age teeth darken owing to the greater amount of reparative dentine.

Patients may have firm ideas about how they want their teeth to look and may bring in photographs of themselves before they lost their teeth. This is often difficult as it is not always possible to reproduce the occlusion and set-up of the natural teeth in dentures. Patients will often choose smaller and lighter teeth than you as a dentist would choose. Outside the mouth, denture teeth look larger than when they are covered with lips and are less well illuminated. The contrast between the colour of denture teeth and the plaster model or the bracket table can be great, and patients should be shown teeth up against their skin or mouth.

In dental terms the shade of restorations is usually described using the Vita shade guide which was originally developed for porcelain shades. Shades are described in terms of hue, chroma, and value. Hue is the colour, chroma is the amount of colour or saturation, and value is the brightness.

In Tilly's case she would probably choose A1 or B1. The Vita shade guide is divided into four groups, A, B, C and D, which each have a specific colour characteristic (or 'hue'):

A: orange-brown
B: yellow
C: grey-brown
D: red.

Each shade letter if further divided into four, designated by a number (e.g. A1, A2, A3, A4). The shade tabs get darker from 1 to 4 (the value decreases) and the chroma or saturation increases from 1 to 4.

Tilly wants A1, while the dentist is convinced that, given her age, the shape of her face and her skin tones, that C2 would give a far more pleasing end result. In the end you agree to compromise on B1.

When the dentures are delivered Tilly is thrilled with her new appearance.

After this, each year in autumn, Tilly reappears. Each year the dentures have either been lost, or broken, or she says they have 'rubbed her gum'. Usually Tilly brings with her a bag full of problem dentures so that she can show the dentist the problems and point out which teeth she liked best in terms of appearance.

Seven years or so pass, with Tilly making annual requests. You notice that she is becoming more and more demanding in her requests. You also notice that her appearance is not as smart as it used to be. She seems not to be looking after herself as she used to.

Your options in the face of Tilly's increasing demands are:
(1) To do nothing and send her away as her 'dental' need is limited.

(2) Continue to make her what she requests even though it is uncertain whether it is in her best dental interests, because she benefits from the visits in other ways.

It would be wrong to continue to make dentures simply because Tilly requests them. The dentist's duty to protect the NHS budget has already been discussed. In light of those comments it was probably wrong to have replaced Tilly's denture in the first instance. She seemed happy with the fit, it was only the size and colour of the teeth that she wanted to change. By providing treatment once for those reasons, it is now more difficult to refuse to treat Tilly once again.

It should have, or ought to have, been obvious to the dentist, at the very latest by Tilly's second set of dentures, that s/he was not dealing with Tilly's problem—be it clinical or psychological. A dentist acting in this way has been remiss in not recognizing her/his failure. Long before the seventh year of replacements the dentist ought to have referred Tilly for a second clinical opinion. Further, if the dentist recognized that Tilly's teeth were not her real problem, the dentist ought to have referred Tilly to her doctor, or at the very least brought the problem to his attention.

(3) Organize some sort of social care for Tilly so that she becomes less dependent on support and company from the dental surgery.

There can be no doubt that if someone has the necessary expertise to assist and help others then they should do so provided that there is no detriment or risk to themselves. However, there is a question of a balance between the help sought and the detriment/risk to the provider. The dentist has the qualifications and experience to provide dental care and consequent to that s/he has a moral duty to help others to the best of her/his ability. Such a moral duty would clearly include established patients but would also extend to include others seeking her/his help.

It may be that the dentist's obligations to Tilly do not stop with dental care. Taking a more holistic approach to patient care, there may be an argument to support the view that the dentist ought to organize some sort of social care for Tilly. However, dentists are not usually in touch with Social Services in the way that their medical colleagues are. Although it would be right and proper, and perhaps a moral obligation for the dentist to seek help for Tilly, Tilly's doctor would be the more appropriate person to do so. The dentist could discharge his obligation by referral to her doctor or informing the doctor of the problems.

TEN YEARS LATER

Ten years later the same dentist receives a telephone call from a local residential home for the elderly, requesting that he visit one of the old ladies who lives at the home.

Treatment at the dental practice or clinic may be ideal but this is not always possible because the patient may require physical assistance and special transport or there may be risks to the patient's physical or emotional well-being.

Home visits are usually necessary when a patient is too ill or disabled or there are carer support problems. Domiciliary visits have the advantage of being more convenient and relaxing for the patient and they also allow an assessment of medications and the level of carer support. However, there are constraints in home visits, mainly relating to the safety of certain clinical procedures. Lighting, seating and suction can be difficult and radiography is practically impossible.

Equipment will depend on the clinical procedures to be carried out, but for any treatment the patient will require suitable seating with head support. This may be achieved by using a high-back chair with additional neck support cushions or a portable back and head rest for a chair, wheelchair, or bed. Good lighting will be required for treatment and this can be difficult in a home. A pen torch, headlight, or intra-oral mirror light may be used.

Restorative treatment will often require a handpiece for caries removal, restoration removal, intra-oral polishing, or for denture adjustment. Portable engines and aspirators are available, if expensive. For denture work a wax heater will be required. Other items to consider are a portable autoclave and a method of disposal of clinical waste.

The dentist duly attends the residence where, on arrival, the matron of the home says that they have a lady suffering from severe senile dementia who appears to be in considerable pain. The matron thinks the pain is emanating from the lady's mouth. Matron informs you that the patient is an insulin-dependent diabetic.

Dementia is a form of physical damage to the brain, which progressively destroys memory and other cognitive abilities. One of the most basic problems associated with patients afflicted with dementia is their inability to describe the presence of symptoms. This clearly makes it very difficult for the clinician to determine the cause of the problem and/or the source of the pain. It is not only that Tilly's dementia may affect her ability to determine the cause of the problem, however, but also that it may even affect her ability to actually perceive the pain she is experiencing. Research has shown that in the moderate stages of cognitive loss associated with the early stages of dementia, people generally respond to painful stimuli and sometimes appear hypersensitive. In later states of dementia, by contrast, patients' responses become more ambiguous and difficult to detect. On the whole, our knowledge of the impact of dementia on pain sensation is not well understood and very little research has been conducted in this area. Consequently, clinical knowledge is poor and there is a paucity of published information available to practitioners.

Diabetes mellitus affects at least 2% of the UK population and up to 6% of the population of the USA. In the older age groups up to 10% may be affected. Diabetes is characterized and diagnosed by a raised blood glucose level, and its severity is largely determined by the degree of the underlying deficiency of insulin action. In diabetics there is an increased susceptibility to infection, poor wound healing, and periodontal disease. Chronic oral infection itself may contribute to raised blood glucose levels. Acute infection in the oral cavity needs specific and aggressive management.

Type 1 diabetes (insulin dependent) most often presents in children or young adults. Characteristic features include sudden onset of symptoms such as thirst, polyuria, weight loss, and lassitude. Life-long insulin injection therapy is required.

Type 2 diabetes (non-insulin dependent) often presents in middle or old age, with a peak onset at 60 years. This type accounts for 80% of all diabetes cases. Clinical management includes diet adjustment as appropriate, oral hypoglycaemic drugs, and in some cases, insulin therapy.

How diabetes affects dental care

Hypoglycaemia is not an uncommon event for diabetics. A fall in blood glucose results in symptoms such as pallor, sweating, confusion, and poor coordination. It is essential to give glucose as if it is untreated at this stage, loss of consciousness may occur. Should this happen then treatment is by intravenous glucose or intramuscular glucagon.

Ketoacidosis follows acute insulin deficiency and is more common in insulin-dependent diabetics than in those who are non-insulin dependent. Serious infections can lead to acute deterioration of diabetes control and ketoacidosis may result from infection unmatched by increased insulin doses. Ketoacidosis requires hospital admission and treatment with intravenous fluids and insulin. Mortality is 5–10% or more in elderly people.

Oral candidosis is more common in diabetic patients, especially if control is poor, and in those wearing dentures. Patients with chronic atrophic candidosis should be advised to use local measures (see earlier).

Periodontal disease: the incidence of loss of periodontal attachment in patients with diabetes is no greater than in the average population if metabolic control and oral hygiene are satisfactory. When metabolic control is poor the diabetic patient will experience greater loss of attachment. Gingivitis has been shown to be more prevalent in those with diabetes despite similar levels of plaque control to non-diabetics.

It is agreed that the dentist will do his best to solve any dental problems and he asks the lady's name. He is told it is Tilly. He enquires as to whether the lady used to attend his surgery but the matron is unsure.

On meeting the patient, the dentist sees at once it is indeed the same Tilly although unsurprisingly there is no glimmer of recognition from her. It is not possible to take a history as Tilly only stares dumbly when you questions are asked.

There seems to be a slight swelling of the right side of Tilly's face. However, when the dentist tries to examine her, Tilly shrinks away and becomes extremely distressed when the dentist continues to attempt the examination. She is in danger of injuring both herself or one of the members of staff. As she yells, the dentist sees that the over-denture abutments are still present but clearly no oral hygiene measures have been undertaken for some time.

Tilly is now in her 70s. She has Alzheimer's. Whilst she would not appear to be refusing treatment, she is not pushing the dentist off, she shrinks away and appears distressed.

Dentists have a duty to act in the best interests of their patients. That is an ethical and legal duty. It is, however, dependent upon the patient's consent to treatment. The dentist's duty does not extend to providing treatment that the patient does not want. The patient's right of self-determination, autonomy, is paramount. That right is supported in law; to carry out treatment without the patient's consent or against their express wishes would be a trespass to their person, a battery more commonly referred to as an assault.

The dentist needs to determine whether Tilly is, by her actions, refusing treatment. All adults are presumed to be competent and to be able to make up their own minds. Without more information it would seem that Tilly is refusing treatment. If that is so then any treatment against Tilly's wishes would be unethical and unlawful. However, the presumption that adults are competent is a rebuttable one and because of that the dentist in this situation, where Alzheimer's is recognized to affect cognitive function, must determine whether Tilly is competent or not.

If Tilly is competent then her refusal is a valid one. The dentist could not ethically or lawfully provide treatment for Tilly even if s/he and/or the nurses felt that it would be in Tilly's best interests. Conversely, if Tilly were considered to be incompetent and the dentist failed to provide any care then not only would this be an unethical position, but it would be unlawful. The current legal duty owed to patients who are unable to decide for themselves is clear:

> In many cases ... it will not only be lawful, for doctors, on the ground of necessity, to operate on or give other medical treatment to adult patients disabled from giving their consent: it will be their common law duty to do so.
>
> [F v. West Berkshire Health Authority (1989) 1 All ER 821 per Lord Brandon at 561]

Upon determining, as is likely, that Tilly is indeed incompetent and her actions cannot be described as a valid refusal but are more of a manifestation of her illness, the dentist will have a duty to do something; to investigate and to alleviate, if required, her apparent suffering.

It is apparent from the scenario that some restraint is going to be required to examine Tilly safely for both her and for the dentist and any support staff. Quite recent law has determined that the use of restraint is a clinical decision and that:

the extent of force or compulsion which may become necessary can only be judged in each individual case and by the health care professionals.

[Re MB (1997) 8 Med LR 217 per Butler-Sloss LJ at 225]

Whether the dentist chooses to use mild physical restraint to examine, or sedation to examine and treat is a clinical decision. It will be based on experience and knowledge. The form of restraint used must be the least intrusive/compulsive which is consistent with safety and success. It may be that the dentist has to progress through mild physical restraint, sedation, and general anaesthesia to achieve that. If the buried upper right third molar which was recognized at Tilly's first presentation is the problem, then the use of general anaesthesia may be justified in the first instance as its removal is unlikely to be achieved with physical restraint or sedation.

You discuss the matter with the matron who tells you that Tilly is sometimes rather aggressive and almost always demanding. She has no known medical problems, other than her diabetes, and she is incontinent because of her Alzheimer's. Matron says there is one daughter who visits occasionally but she is not aware of any other living relatives. Matron is also aware that Tilly has been a widow for many years.

All the staff at the home have noticed Tilly clutching at the right side of her face in increasing desperation, sometimes in tears. Unfortunately, Tilly's communicative powers are so diminished that she is unable to tell anyone what her problem is, although sometimes the desperation in her eyes is all too obvious.

Diagnosis

Tilly appears to have a swelling, very probably of dental origin. On consulting Tilly's previous notes the dentist becomes aware that a buried UR8 may well be the cause of the problem. However, diagnosis without examination is problematic.

Treatment options

1. Do nothing.
2. Forcibly examine the patient, perhaps under sedation, with a view to treating any problems, if appropriate, with antibiotics and pain killers.
3. Organize examination under general anaesthetic, plus extraction of UR8.

1. Doing nothing is not an option in this case as the patient is in pain. In fact, it would be illogical for a dentist to dismiss this senile lady as uncooperative and therefore untreatable, as every dentist is legally bound to do their best for a patient. This is the dentist's 'duty of care'.
2. If the patient would accept intravenous sedation and could be sedated to an extent whereby treatment could be carried out then this is a viable option. However, there would be no way of knowing what procedure you would end up doing and therefore no way of judging whether or not it will be possible. That is, it might be possible to remove one mobile,

periodontally involved tooth under local anaesthesia under sedation but if Tilly's pain turned out to be due to something more sinister, requiring a general anaesthetic then the sedation would have been undertaken to no good purpose, other than to establish the diagnosis.

3. In order that all of Tilly's dental problems are dealt with (as clearly she will not cooperate for treatment in the future) and because you are aware of the presence of the UR8 and the lower canine abutments (which you think are of very poor prognosis due to the lack of oral hygiene), all of which can be removed under general anaesthetic, it may be necessary for Tilly to have this treatment done. The benefits must be weighed against the risks, which in a frail old lady are considerable, and the issue of consent must be carefully managed.

Option (3) is best if you suspect that Tilly has anything wrong with her mouth which you could not treat under sedation and local anaesthesia.

BIBLIOGRAPHY

Bell GW, Large DM, Barclay SC. Oral health care in diabetes mellitus. *Dental Update* 1999; **26**(8): 322–330.

Bergandal B. The relative importance of tooth loss and denture wearing. *Community Dental Health* 1989; **6**: 103–111.

Devlin H. *Prosthodontics: a Case-based Learning Approach*. Springer: Berlin, 2001.

Ehas AC, Sheiham A. The relationship between satisfaction with mouth, and, number position and condition of teeth. *Journal of Oral Rehabilitation* 1999; **26**: 53–71.

Ettinger RL. Clinical decision making in the dental treatment of the elderly. *Gerondentology* 1984; **3**: 157–165.

Gift HC, Atchison KA. Oral health, health and health-related quality of life. *Medical Care* 1995; **33**: 57–77.

Humphris GM. Communicating with patients about oral cancer, *Continuing Professional Development in Dentistry* 2001; **2**(1): 26–29.

Humphris GM, Ireland RS, Field EA. Immediate knowledge increase from an oral cancer information leaflet in patients attending a primary care facility: a randomized controlled trial. *Oral Oncology* 2001; **37**(1): 99–102.

Kay EJ, Nuttall NM. *Clinical Decision Making. An Art or a Science*. BDJ Books: London, 1997.

Kelly M, Steele J, Nuttall N, Bradnock G, Morris J, Nunn J, Pine C, Pitts N, Treasure E, White D. *Adult Dental Health Survey. Oral Health in the United Kingdom, 1998*, p. 557. HMSO: London, 2000.

Leake JL, Hawkins R, Locker D. Social and functional impact of reduced posterior dental units in older adults. *Journal of Oral Rehabilitation* 1994; **21**: 1–10.

Locker D. Does dental care improve oral health of the elderly. *Community Dental Health* 2001; **18**: 7–15.

Locker D, Clarke M, Payne B. Self-perceived oral health status, psychological well being and life satisfaction in an older adult population. *Journal of Dental Research* 2000; **79**: 970–975.

Mechanic D. Energising trends in the application of the social sciences in health and medicine. *Social Science and Medicine* 1995; **40**: 1491.

O'Reilly PG, Claffey NM. A history of oral sepsis as a cause of disease. *Periodontology* 2000; **23**: 13–18.

Reisine S, Locker D. Social, psychological and economic impacts of oral conditions and treatments. In: Cohen LK, Gift HC (eds) *Disease Prevention and Oral Health Promotion. Socio-Dental Sciences in Action*, pp. 33–71. Munksgaard: Copenhagen.

Sheiham A, Goog SH. The psychosocial impact of dental diseases on individuals and communities. *Journal of Behavioral Medicine* 1981; **4**: 257–272.

Smith JM, Sheiham A. How dental conditions handicap the elderly. *Community Dentistry and Oral Epidemiology* 1979; **12**: 305–310.

Strauss RP, Hunt RJ. Understanding the value of teeth to older adults: influences on the quality of life. *Journal of the American Dental Association* 1993; **124**: 105–110.

Walker EA, Milgrom PM, Weinstein P, Getz T, Richardson R. Assessing abuse and neglect and dental fear in women. *Journal of the American Dental Association* 1996; **127**(4): 485–490.

Josh presented first at the age of 4 years. His grandmother attended with him. She reported that his father was in prison and that his mother could not cope with Josh or his two younger sisters due to her drug problems. His grandmother dearly loved the children but clearly found it very difficult to deal with all three of them. Josh was apparently fit and well but had been awake for three nights screaming with toothache. He was somewhat disruptive in the surgery, objecting to almost any request made to him. After much persuasion and some bribery Josh allowed a very brief examination of his teeth and was persuaded to have lateral oblique radiographs taken (easier than bitewings for less than cooperative children).

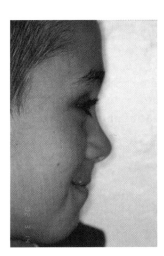 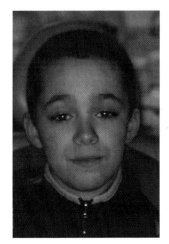

Josh

How do you help children to become cooperative?
What techniques can be used?

The (albeit) brief examination of Josh's mouth revealed that every tooth was decayed with the upper incisors being decayed/eroded to gingival level. The majority of the molar teeth were pulpally involved and the teeth were covered with plaque.

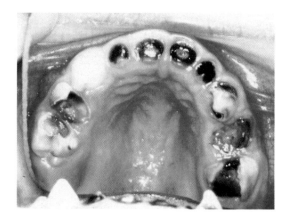

Gross caries in deciduous dentition

Diagnosis

Josh's problems were as listed below:

1. Gross caries in the majority of dentition.
2. 'Nursing-bottle caries' in anterior teeth.
3. Very poor oral hygiene.
4. Poor cooperation.
5. Social circumstances not conducive to oral health or normal development.
6. Highly cariogenic diet.

The treatment options for Josh at this stage were very limited. Extraction under general anaesthetic (GA) of all carious deciduous teeth was planned.

Were any other treatment plans viable?

What are the steps when planning treatment for children?

Josh's grandmother was given preventive advice, a further prevention appointment was made and extraction of the deciduous dentition under general anaesthesia was arranged.

Josh's grandmother was worried when she was told that for a general anaesthetic written parental consent was required. She stated that Josh's mother or father would not be able to attend (she did not specify why). On the day of the anaesthetic, Josh attended with a social worker who produced a document which he said allowed him to act 'in loco parentis'. It was he who signed Josh's consent form.

Could Josh's grandmother sign the consent?

Is written consent always necessary for a GA?

Josh did not attend for his post-GA prevention appointments.

Can children eat without any teeth?

Why did Josh not attend for his appointments?

Four years later: Aged 8, Josh attended complaining about the 'big black holes' in his front teeth. He claimed this was his only problem.

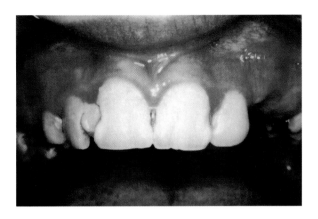

Immature central incisors with large cavities

On this occasion, Josh attended again with his grandmother. She, unlike Josh, claimed that he had experienced pain from a tooth at the back on the right and that it hurt Josh when he chewed. He was, despite some initial bravado and the declaration that 'I'm not having no needles', reasonably cooperative. He allowed examination of his mouth although a careful 'tell–show–do' regime was required to maintain his limited trust. He seemed to respond well to being talked to as if he were a 'tough' teenager. It was eventually possible, at this visit, to take bitewings and a dental panoramic tomographic (DPT) radiograph.

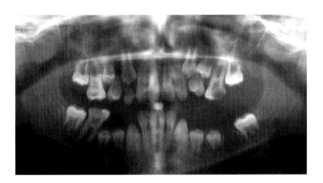

Carious dentition in 8–9 year old

Josh's examination revealed large cavities in all four first permanent molars. The upper incisors all had mesial and distal cavities with UR2, UL1 having deep lesions which radiographically appeared to be close to the pulp. Lower central incisors also had cavities. The cavity in LR6 was deep and there were radio-graphic signs of periapical pathology. Josh's oral hygiene was very poor with plaque covering two-thirds of all teeth.

Josh denied having had any toothache except from his front tooth. His main concern was the black hole in his 2|. At age 8, Josh seemed incredibly concerned about his appearance.

Does the way a child looks matter?

Diagnosis

Josh's dental problems were, therefore, at age 8:

1. Caries in six incisor teeth and all four first permanent molars with periapical involvement LR6.
2. Very poor oral hygiene.
3. Extremely high caries rate.
4. Poor aesthetic appearance anteriorly.
5. Poor cooperation, particularly regarding local anaesthetic (LA).

This case left the dentist in an extreme treatment planning dilemma.

If cooperation for LA could be gained, UR6, UL6, LL6 could perhaps be restored, but of course unless a preventive regime was followed (which given past experience seemed highly unlikely) the long-term prognosis for the first permanent molars was poor, given the incredibly high caries rate (the 6s had, at this stage, only been erupted for 2 years and yet one already had caries to the pulp). It was also possible that the experience of having these teeth restored might reduce cooperation further. In addition, Josh's chief motivator for attendance seemed to be the appearance of the anterior teeth. Again, if LA could be used these teeth were restorable, although root canal therapy of UR1, UL2 in the near future seemed likely to be necessary. The question of whether Josh would continue to attend for complex treatment involving RCTs therefore had to be taken into consideration.

Treatment options

1. Extract all carious teeth under GA. Fit temporary denture and offer prevention for teeth still to erupt. This option would improve Josh's appearance, yet to fit a denture prior to the eruption of the remaining permanent teeth makes this plan less than ideal.
2. Gain cooperation for LA: restore anteriors, restore first permanent molars, extract LR6 LA/GA.
3. Temporize all carious teeth. Gain cooperation for LA. Commence prevention. If the first two items are achieved, make a definitive treatment plan.

None of these treatment options seemed to offer Josh either immediate relief of symptoms, long-term improvement of appearance, or the likelihood of good oral health in the future. To commit an 8-year-old to dentures could potentially be extremely damaging to both Josh's attitude and his oral health.

After long discussion with Josh and his grandmother, it was decided that the third option would be attempted under inhalation sedation (IHS). Josh was initially adamant that he would not have either the sedation or an injection. However, after explanation of the alternative treatment plans, he agreed to try sedation (although not an injection).

Treatment

At the first sedation visit Josh again stated, quite aggressively, that he would not have 'a needle' and that he did not trust the dentist not to put him to sleep with the sedation.

A bizarre, but in the end helpful, intervention from Grandma was useful at this point. She told Josh that the 'happy air' would be just like one of Uncle Hal's 'funny cigarettes'. This seemed to soothe Josh. He appeared to then think that the sedation would be 'cool' and cooperated brilliantly.

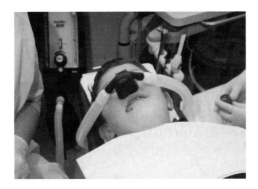

Relative analgesia on a child

Is it legal for a dentist to ignore information about drug use?

The next issue was local anaesthesia. Josh was too suspicious and 'street smart' to be hoodwinked by the subtle approaches which often work with other children (it's just a cold spray, etc). Thus, the dentist explained that the teeth could not be 'mended' without it hurting him unless Josh had an injection. Still Josh was adamant that he was not having 'the needle'.

At this point, following to some extent Grandma's lead, the dentist pointed out that someone 'cool' enough to have a doubly pierced ear [Josh] could not possibly be so scared of a tiny injection. Josh then agreed to the injection so long as it would not hurt.

From this point the visits went as follows:

1. First visit: Inhalation sedation, acclimatization, and oral hygiene.

This was extremely effective with Josh sedating deeply on 20% N₂O. His teeth were polished, much praise was given and Josh thoroughly enjoyed the visit, especially the 'happy air'. He was happy then to come again for his front tooth to be filled under local anaesthesia.

Why is it important to try to make children happy about attending the dentist?

It was explained to Josh that one cannot put white fillings in teeth with dirty gums. The plaque was demonstrated to Josh—who then proclaimed people with plaque in their mouths to be 'disgusting'. He agreed to brush regularly to make his gums healthy enough for his fillings to be done. The dentist wrote a 'pledge' about oral hygiene in Josh's notes, which Josh signed. He responded well to this 'grown-up' agreement. At the next visit his mouth, though far from spotless, was far far cleaner.

What makes people behave in healthy or unhealthy ways?

2. Second visit: Josh accepted sedation and local anaesthesia. Much was made of how 'cool' he was.

Is telling someone they are 'cool' an appropriate reward for good behaviour?

UR1, UR2 were excavated and dressed with glass ionomer cement (GIC). This semi-temporary dressing, though far from being a perfect restorative treatment, fulfilled Josh's desire to radically improve his appearance. Such dressings are also quicker and more easily achieved than composite restorations. The vitality of UR2 was tested with a view to long-term monitoring prior to definitive treatment. Josh was delighted with his achievements and the results.

Is filling anterior teeth with GIC appropriate?

3. Third visit: LL1, LR1 were restored with composite under IHS and local anaesthesia.
4. Fourth visit: UL1, UL2 were restored with composite under IHS and local anaesthesia.

   Josh was then aged 10. Josh was then given a general anaesthetic appointment for extraction of his first permanent molars. It may have been possible to restore at least some of these teeth, but LR6 required extraction and because of the poor long-term prognosis of the other 6s, it was felt to be in Josh's best interests to remove all four teeth.

Why extract four permanent molars when only one is unrestorable?

Josh's mother and father attended with him for the GA appointment.

Between the visits described above, there were many cancelled and broken appointments. This, the Grandma revealed, was because Josh was so often in youth court. He was playing truant, staying out until after midnight, had been arrested for burning cars and was not attending school.

Can the dentist refuse to continue to treat Josh?

Three years later: Josh attended again, aged 13, accompanied by his mother. He said that food is getting 'stuck' in his back teeth. When asked if Josh was now attending school, his mother stated that he was not and that he had twice absconded from home and lived rough for five days, one of these occasions being very recent. Josh's mum said that he would eat very little except 'custard cream' biscuits which he ate at the rate of three to four packets per day.

On examination (for which Josh was very cooperative without the need for sedation) the anterior 'semi-permanent' restorations were still in place. Fur-

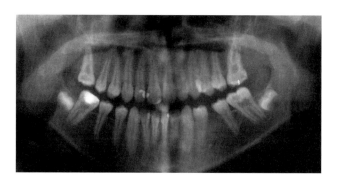

DPT of Josh aged 13 years

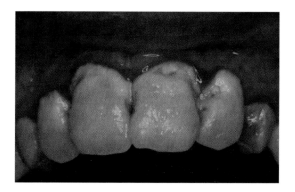

Poor oral hygiene

ther cavities had developed in LL1, LR1. The second permanent molars were fully erupted, as were the canines and premolars. Visual signs of caries were seen in all four second permanent molars.

Radiographs showed very deep cavities in LR7, LL7 and cavities in UR7, UL7. The oral hygiene was very poor.

Treatment options

1. Extract all second permanent molars under general anaesthetic. Preventive regime. Restorations as required, if attendance permitted. Extract anterior teeth under LA/sedation when there are signs or symptoms.

2. Restore UR7, UL7 under IHS and LA. Extract LL7, LR7 under IHS and LA. Extract anterior teeth when there are signs or symptoms and supply partial denture.

3. Extract all remaining teeth and provide F/F denture.

Once again, Josh had provided a treatment planning dilemma of the most extreme kind. Any faith in his ability to maintain any kind of oral health regime had clearly been misplaced (this was obviously not Josh's fault, more the fault of his circumstances), and yet to remove further problems by providing dentures for a still-growing jaw seemed almost cruel.

Why is it so difficult to make Josh's mouth healthy?

The dentist opted for the first of the treatment plans, i.e. extraction of all second permanent molars under general anaesthetic; however, when this was discussed, Josh asked whether anyone ever died under general anaesthetic. The dentist attempted to describe the probability of such an event using the analogy of one person out of two football stadia full of people. Josh insisted that he might be that one person who was unlucky. In fact, his words were: 'knowing me, I'll be that one'. The dentist could sort of see his point!

Thus, the issue of the personal autonomy of children and consent made it necessary to change the treatment plan to option 2.

Is Josh able to refuse an anaesthetic if his mother and the dentist think it in his interest?

At the next visit, at which UR7, UL7 were to be restored under LA and sedation, Josh was accompanied by his aunt. She explained that he was now living with her and was attending a new school, which catered particularly for boys with Josh's kinds of difficulties. She was very concerned about the need for extractions of LL7, LR7 and stated that it was her and Josh's wish that he kept his teeth if at all possible. The very poor state of and prognosis for the teeth were explained. Also Josh was anxious about the extractions. Given that the treatment plan was far from ideal, the dentist agreed to investigate the teeth and restore them if at all possible.

Is it acceptable for a dentist to choose a treatment plan which he knows is not ideal?

On examining Josh's mouth, the dentist noted that it was considerably cleaner. The aunt said that now that Josh had a more settled life, he would be taking better care of his mouth and that his diet was now much better.

The dentist then proceeded to open the UL7, which required antibiotic steroid dressing as it was cariously exposed.

What effect do antibiotic steroid dressings have on pulpal tissue?

The dilemma regarding extraction thus remained.

Josh was not seen again until years later.

Six years later, aged 19, Josh attended with severe pain in the lower left quadrant. The anterior teeth all had large open cavities. Josh looked thin and unwell.

On questioning, he admitted that he had been a heroin addict from aged 16. Recently (in the past 6 months) he had been treated with methadone in an attempt to break his habit.

What is the significance of Josh's methadone programme?

Josh tells the dentist that he has his own house which he shares with his 17-year-old girlfriend and his 1-year-old son, whom he clearly adores. He was concerned about the rapidly deteriorating appearance of his mouth and of course the almost intolerable pain he was suffering.

When a medical history was taken, Josh said that he had been seriously ill with liver disease. He had been told this was due to using dirty needles to inject. He was also HIV positive.

What should a dentist ask about in a medical history?

Are there any particular difficulties in providing dental treatment for drug addicts?

What precautions should be taken if a patient has a blood-borne virus?

After taking a careful medical history from Josh, an intra-oral radiographic examination revealed the following:

1. Gross caries of all remaining teeth.
2. Pulpal involvement of badly broken down upper incisors, second permanent molars, and lower centrals.
3. Periapical pathology of LR7.
4. Draining sinuses UR2, UL1.
5. 'High-risk' patient.

The prognosis for the remaining teeth is extremely poor. The chance of Josh attending regularly for root treatments/crowns was, in the dentist's view, zero, even if this were a viable treatment option. Doing nothing was also not an option due to Josh's severe pain.

Can the dentist refuse to treat Josh?

Thus, this seemed to be one of those extremely rare cases whereby clearance of the remaining teeth and provision of a denture appeared to be the only sensible option.

Could the dentist have taken better actions/decisions earlier which would have avoided this poor outcome?

JOSH: A LAD WITH PROBLEMS

Josh presented first at the age of 4 years. His grandmother attended with him. She reported that his father was in prison and that his mother could not cope with Josh or his two younger sisters due to her drug problems. His grandmother dearly loved the children but clearly found it very difficult to deal with all three of them. Josh was apparently fit and well but had been awake for three nights screaming with toothache. He was somewhat disruptive in the surgery, objecting to almost any request made to him. After much persuasion and some bribery Josh allowed a very brief examination of his teeth and was persuaded to have lateral oblique radiographs taken (easier than bitewings for less than cooperative children).

It is useful to think of all 'difficult' patients as 'pre-cooperative'. This focuses the dentist's mind on the fact that all patients can (with management appropriate to the individual's circumstances) become cooperative.

Several techniques are useful, but with children particularly it is helpful to keep in mind their stage of development and their ability to cope with new situations and strange people. Generally speaking, children who have only experienced adults as helpful, kind and interested beings tend to accept explanation and novel procedures more easily than those for whom strangers may be potentially 'dangerous'—i.e. may separate them from their family, may ignore their wishes, or may even hurt them. Children who repeatedly indulge in disruptive and attention-seeking behaviour (often perceived as plain naughtiness) often have their behaviours reinforced because it almost invariably gains adult attention. Such children are more time-consuming and difficult to deal with than those whose lives have taught them that 'being good' and going along with adult plans often brings pleasurable experiences.

The 'tell–show–do' technique is a basic 'must-do' when dealing with any child. This involves firstly an explanation, in words which the child understands, then a demonstration (either on a model or on the child's hand, or even the dentist's hand) and lastly the action is undertaken. Children's natural curiosity and interest in the world around them with its ever-available new experiences almost invariably makes this technique at least partially successful.

What is particularly important with very disruptive children, who simply do not wish dentistry to proceed (as opposed to them being frightened), is to try very hard to ignore non-desired behaviours and to positively reward any progress towards the desired goal. Thus, any behaviour, such as getting on the chair, opening the mouth, staying open when asked, MUST be met with huge praise and hearty encouragement.

Other techniques include forced choices. In this technique, one can give the child choices, all of which lead to the desired goal. A closed question is asked in which all the available responses lead to the outcome the dentist wants. For example, if a child is showing signs of not sitting in the chair, a choice can be offered as to which side to get on it from. Children, even the most hostile and recalcitrant, are often so surprised to be given the seemingly grown-up role of making decisions for themselves that they will take one of the choices offered (this side, or that side) even though, in actual fact, doing so leads them to do something against which they had set their minds. The point is, the option of 'No' as a potential answer is not given, as in: 'Will you sit in the chair'. A further example would be achieving a 'polish' by offering the child 'top teeth or bottom teeth first'. Praise for all cooperation is still essential but this 'choosing' technique is almost always extremely effective.

Telling children how fantastic, grown up, or better than 'all the other boys and girls' they are offers them the necessary feeling of achievement. Once small steps have been achieved, most children, in order to gain the praise and attention of other people, will go on to take bigger and bolder steps towards the goal.

It is important at each visit to have a clear goal, or achievement, for the child. This serves two purposes. It gives the dentist a sense of direction and allows each visit to end with praise and reinforcement for the child's achievements. If a child easily reaches the goal, the visit should end. Pushing a child for more and more cooperation will lead to their refusing at some point. This means the visit ends on a low, rather than high point, which will undermine the child's experience of dentistry as something positive.

The (albeit) brief examination of Josh's mouth revealed that every tooth was decayed with the upper incisors being decayed/eroded to gingival level. The majority of the molar teeth were pulpally involved and the teeth were covered with plaque.

Diagnosis

Josh's problems were as listed below:
1. Gross caries in the majority of dentition.
2. 'Nursing-bottle caries' in anterior teeth.
3. Very poor oral hygiene.
4. Poor cooperation.
5. Social circumstances not conducive to oral health or normal development.
6. Highly cariogenic diet.

The treatment options for Josh at this stage were very limited. Extraction under general anaesthetic (GA) of all carious deciduous teeth was planned.

In children with acute pain, in whom many teeth are carious with pulpal involvement, there is little alternative to general anaesthesia and extraction of all the teeth likely to be causing the pain, plus any others with poor prognosis. In children such as Josh, consideration of space loss due to early loss of deciduous molars is not of importance. The treatment plan should involve:
1. pain relief,
2. prevention,
3. pursuit of cooperation,
4. perfect dentistry.

Such a regime should always be followed, as attempting to achieve anything in any other order is doomed to failure. Unfortunately, in many cases, once pain is relieved, the social circumstances of dentally needy children often lead to poor attendance.

Josh's grandmother was given preventive advice, a further prevention appointment was made and extraction of the deciduous dentition under general anaesthesia was arranged.

Josh's grandmother was worried when she was told that for a general anaesthetic written parental consent was required. She stated that Josh's mother or
father would not be able to attend (she did not specify why). On the day of the
anaesthetic, Josh attended with a social worker who produced a document which
he said allowed him to act 'in loco parentis'. It was he who signed Josh's consent
form.

Josh's family are clearly in difficulties. His father is in prison and his mother has
a drug problem. He is 4 and has two younger sisters. While he and his sisters
live with his grandmother they are almost certain to be under the care of the
Local Authority, the grandmother simply being a foster carer rather than
a legal guardian. In such circumstances the Local Authority will have an
Order of the Court granting it parental responsibility. It is unlikely that the
grandmother will have parental responsibility.

Josh first attended the dentist with his grandmother for the examination.
The issue of lawful consent is, therefore, worthy of discussion.

At the first attendance Josh was in pain. It was important to examine him at
the very least. In such circumstances the Children Act 1989 provides for the
grandmother's 'consent'. Section 3(5) states that a person who does not have
parental responsibility for a child but has care of the child should do what is
reasonable in all the circumstances of the case for the purpose of safeguarding
or promoting the child's welfare. Thus, in these circumstances, the dentist
would be permitted to carry out an examination in the absence of consent,
under the common law doctrine of necessity and that examination would be
lawful provided that it was in Josh's best interests and that it was a reasonable
thing to do in the circumstances.

On return for the general anaesthetic Josh is accompanied by his social
worker. In respect of the consent required for the provision of general anaesthesia the requirement of a written consent is not a legal issue. It is a requirement set down by the General Dental Council. Insofar as the law is concerned
there is no requirement for consent to be written. Further, written consent is
not conclusive that consent was in fact given but merely evidence that it may
have been. In the light of what has been said in the preceding paragraph the
social worker is an appropriate person to give lawful consent.

There may be an issue here in respect of Josh's medical history. The social
worker may not be aware of Josh's medical history. This may be a matter for the
anaesthetist rather than the dentist.

Josh did not attend for his post-GA prevention appointments.

It is surprising how well children who are rendered edentulous cope. They seem
able to eat almost all foods within a modern diet and although the treatment
given to Josh is far from ideal, relief of his pain and avoidance of further anaesthesia (which would be the consequence in a child with such a high caries
rate if any carious teeth had been left *in situ*) indicated that this radical and
destructive treatment was still the treatment of choice.

Clearly, for families who live in fairly extreme social circumstances, attendance at the dentist is often difficult and perhaps may not be a priority. There is also a popular population belief that the deciduous dentition, since it is lost anyway, is expendable and of relative unimportance in terms of perceived health. In Josh's case, he was asked to attend for preventive advice when he had no teeth. Whilst dentists might understand that this is a sensible way forward and in Josh's best interests, it is perhaps not difficult to see that both Josh, his parents, and grandmother would see little point in attending when there were no problems AND no teeth! Treatment planning must always take account of how the patient and his family perceive their health-care needs, rather than focusing simply on ideal clinical treatments. If a dentist simply imposes his views and values on people, they will simply not 'comply' with treatment or appointments. As they see it, doing so does not benefit them in any way. Health and oral health are subjective experiences, not something which one person (a dentist) can give to, or impose upon, another (a patient).

Four years later: Aged 8, Josh attended complaining about the 'big black holes' in his front teeth. He claimed this was his only problem.

On this occasion, Josh attended again with his grandmother. She, unlike Josh, claimed that he had experienced pain from a tooth at the back on the right and that it hurt Josh when he chewed. He was, despite some initial bravado and the declaration that 'I'm not having no needles', reasonably cooperative. He allowed examination of his mouth although a careful 'tell–show–do' regime was required to maintain his limited trust. He seemed to respond well to being talked to as if he were a 'tough' teenager. It was eventually possible, at this visit, to take bitewings and a dental panoramic tomographic (DPT) radiograph.

Josh's examination revealed large cavities in all four first permanent molars. 21|12 all had mesial and distal cavities with 2|, |1 having deep lesions which radiographically appeared to be close to the pulp. 1/1 also had cavities. The cavity in 6| was deep and there were radiographic signs of periapical pathology. Josh's oral hygiene was very poor with plaque covering two-thirds of all teeth.

Josh denied having had any toothache except from his front tooth. His main concern was the black hole in his 2|. At age 8, Josh seemed incredibly concerned about his appearance.

It is not surprising that children are so concerned with 'appearance' and 'attractiveness'. They learn this from adults. Table 1 briefly lists just some of the studies conducted on adults, which have demonstrated some important interpersonal and social consequences associated with appearance, especially with 'facial attractiveness'.

More specifically related to children, however, numerous studies have shown links between appearance and popularity amongst peers. A large-scale study of both American and Japanese school children of varying ages examined their evaluations of the reasons why certain children were excluded

Table 1. Studies exploring the effect of facial attractiveness on social interaction

Study 1: Male and female experimenters approached students on a college campus and tried to get them to sign a petition. The more attractive the experimenters were, the more signatures they were able to get

Study 2: Texas judges set lower bail and imposed smaller fines on suspects who were rated as attractive rather than unattractive

Study 3: The 'baby-face bias' also influences the outcome of court cases. In a US study, baby-faced defendants were much more frequently found innocent in cases involving intentional wrongdoing than were mature-faced defendants. However, there was no difference between baby-faced and mature-faced defendants in cases involving negligence. This effect was highly significant even when statistical means were used to equate baby-faced and mature-faced defendants for age, sex, and various other factors that could have affected the judge's decision

Study 4: Mothers of highly attractive babies were observed to be more attentive, affectionate, and playful in their interactions than mothers with less attractive infants

Study 5: Across occupational groups in the US and Canada, attractive men and women earn more money than others who are comparable except for being less attractive in their appearance

from peer groups. One of the most common reasons given was 'having an unconventional appearance'. Research on bullying also shows that physical appearance plays an important role, including any facial or dental anomalies. Teasing related to dental appearance appears to be particularly hurtful. Studies of paediatric cancer patients have also shown that they often have problems in social and psychological adjustment related to their appearance. In one study, children recorded peer popularity ratings for photographs of children with and without hair. Children gave significantly lower popularity ratings to photographs of bald children than to those with hair. Another study found some important differences in gender and race with regard to the relationship between self-perception and peer acceptance. For instance, it was found that the relationship between peer acceptance and perceived physical appearance was significantly stronger for Black boys in comparison with White boys and girls of either race.

One interesting study investigated the extent to which the interaction between minor physical anomalies and family adversity predicted violent and non-violent delinquency during adolescence. This study looked at 170 adolescent boys from lower socioeconomic backgrounds in Montreal. It found that minor physical anomalies, especially related to the mouth, were significantly associated with an increased risk of violent delinquency during adolescence. This association held even when the effects of childhood physical aggression and family adversity were accounted for. However, similar findings were not established for non-violent delinquency. The study concluded that children with a higher count of physical anomalies, especially of the mouth, could be more difficult to socialize for a number of different, additive reasons.

Diagnosis

Josh's dental problems were, therefore, at age 8
1. Caries six incisors and all four first permanent molars with periodontal involvement LR6.
2. Very poor oral hygiene.
3. Extremely high caries rate.
4. Poor aesthetic appearance anteriorly.
5. Poor cooperation, particularly regarding local anaesthetic (LA).
    This case left the dentist in an extreme treatment planning dilemma.

If cooperation for LA could be gained, UR6, UL6, LL6 could perhaps be restored, but of course unless a preventive regime was followed (which given past experience seemed highly unlikely) the long-term prognosis for the first permanent molars was poor, given the incredibly high caries rate (the 6s had, at this stage, only been erupted for 2 years and yet one already had caries to the pulp). It was also possible that the experience of having these teeth restored might reduce cooperation further. In addition, Josh's chief motivator for attendance seemed to be the appearance of the anterior teeth. Again, if LA could be used these teeth were restorable, although root canal therapy of UR1, UL2 in the near future seemed likely to be necessary. The question of whether Josh would continue to attend for complex treatment involving RCTs therefore had to be taken into consideration.

Treatment options
1. Extract all carious teeth under GA. Fit temporary denture and offer prevention for teeth still to erupt. This option would improve Josh's appearance, yet to fit a denture prior to the eruption of the remaining permanent teeth makes this plan less than ideal.
2. Gain cooperation for LA: restore anteriors, restore first permanent molars, extract LR6, LA/GA.
3. Temporize all carious teeth. Gain cooperation for LA. Commence prevention. If the first two items are achieved, make a definitive treatment plan.

None of these treatment options seemed to offer Josh either immediate relief of symptoms, long-term improvement of appearance, or the likelihood of good oral health in the future. Yet to commit an 8-year-old to dentures could potentially be extremely damaging to both Josh's attitude and his oral health.

After long discussion with Josh and his grandmother, it was decided that the third option would be attempted under inhalation sedation (IHS). Josh was initially adamant that he would not have either the sedation or an injection. However, after explanation of the alternative treatment plans, he agreed to try sedation (although not an injection).

Treatment

At the first sedation visit Josh again stated, quite aggressively, that he would not have 'a needle' and that he did not trust the dentist not to put him to sleep with the sedation.

A bizarre, but in the end helpful, intervention from Grandma was useful at this point. She told Josh that the 'happy air' would be just like one of Uncle Hal's 'funny cigarettes'. This seemed to soothe Josh. He appeared to then think that the sedation would be 'cool' and cooperated brilliantly.

There can be no doubt that the dentist cannot ignore and not act on what s/he has heard. As a health-care professional it would part of her/his duty of care for Josh, to have concern for his general health and welfare, not simply for his teeth. In the first instance the dentist may consider contacting Josh's general medical practitioner. If this is not possible for some reason, then the Local Authority. Such disclosure will raise many complex issues in respect of Josh's care and place of residence but these are issues to be decided by a fully informed court, it would not be for the dentist to prejudge any such issues by non-disclosure.

The next issue was local anaesthesia. Josh was too suspicious and 'street smart' to be hoodwinked by the subtle approaches which often work with other children (it's just a cold spray, etc). Thus, the dentist explained that the teeth could not be 'mended' without it hurting him unless Josh had an injection. Still Josh was adamant that he was not having 'the needle'.

At this point, following to some extent Grandma's lead, the dentist pointed out that someone 'cool' enough to have a doubly pierced ear [Josh] could not possibly be so scared of a tiny injection. Josh then agreed to the injection so long as it would not hurt.

From this point the visits went as follows:

1. First visit: Inhalation sedation, acclimatization, and oral hygiene.

This was extremely effective with Josh sedating deeply on 20% N_2O. His teeth were polished, much praise was given and Josh thoroughly enjoyed the visit, especially the 'happy air'. He was happy then to come again for his front tooth to be filled under local anaesthesia.

Children who are only taken to the dentist when they have trouble, i.e. experience pain from their teeth, have greater numbers of decayed and/or filled teeth than children who attend for regular dental check-ups. Two-thirds of 8-year-old children who only attend the dentist when they experience symptoms have active decay, whilst in children who attend the dentist more frequently, only about a third can be expected to have tooth decay.

It was explained to Josh that one cannot put white fillings in teeth with dirty gums. The plaque was demonstrated to Josh—who then proclaimed people with plaque in their mouths to be 'disgusting'. He agreed to brush regularly to make his gums healthy enough for his fillings to be done. The dentist wrote a 'pledge' about oral hygiene in Josh's notes, which Josh signed. He responded well to this 'grown-up' agreement. At the next visit his mouth, though far from spotless, was far far cleaner.

One of the main factors associated with whether or not we engage in various health behaviours is whether or not we perceive ourselves to be in control. Even, perhaps especially, children feel this. Perception of control means the subjective determination of the ability to determine or influence something. In this case, this 'something' is Josh's ability to influence his own oral hygiene. Living in a family environment where he has very little control over what is happening around him, Josh can gain a strong sense of achievement from his relationship with the dentist and perhaps from making an effort to try and influence his own health in some small way. The very fact that the dentist is taking him seriously and engaging with him on this issue may in itself increase his sense of self-confidence and self-worth. In effect, what the dentist is doing here is increasing Josh's sense of control and thus making it more likely that he will engage in the oral health plan necessary to improve his dentition.

An important psychological theory to consider here is 'social learning theory'. This theory proposes that, in any given situation, the likelihood that a person will engage in a particular behaviour (or set of behaviours) is a function of two things: (1) the person's expectancy that the behaviour will lead to a particular outcome in that situation and (2) the value of the outcome to the person in that situation. It is very important, therefore, that in Josh's case any initial behaviour he performs in relation to improved oral health is properly rewarded (and thus reinforced) by the dentist. This might include strong praise and further emphasis on the fact that he's a 'tough teenager'. With most children, stickers and certificates normally go down very well—but given Josh's 'streetwise' persona, he may consider this a bit 'beneath' him. If relevant 'rewards' are provided from the very beginning, Josh will anticipate such praise in the future, and internally, this may provide him with a stronger sense of self-esteem and control. These positive internal feelings will obviously make it more likely that he will engage in orally healthy behaviour in the future.

Of course, the main problem is that such 'expectancies' are not strictly situation specific. The individual tends, through a variety of learning experiences, to develop 'generalized expectancies' that cut across different situations. If the child is from an unstable and unpredictable environment, his/her expectations may be very low and s/he may not believe that they will be 'rewarded' in any way for any behaviour. In such situations we see the antithesis of 'learned control'. Instead, we have a feeling of helplessness—developed in another theory called 'learned helplessness'. This is a situation in which a person comes to believe that outcomes are not at all contingent on his/her behaviour. This can obviously have rather negative motivational, emotional, and behavioural consequences. Feeling helpless is associated with a feeling of incompetence and non-self-efficacy. People who feel helpless are unlikely to engage in 'positive' health behaviours and will also easily abandon behaviours that have a 'positive' effect on health because they feel they have no control over their life anyway.

It is perhaps not surprising that there is a strong link between helplessness and depression. In turn, depression is associated with 'negative' health behaviours such as substance abuse and attempted suicides.

2. Second visit: Josh accepted sedation and local anaesthesia. Much was made of how 'cool' he was.

It is important to remember that no two people are alike and something which would act as praise for one child may be irrelevant to another. For example, being thought of as 'clever' is not particularly important to Josh, neither is being 'liked'. But being thought of as 'cool' is important to him in the context of his own life. 'Cool' is what he aspires to. Thus, when seeking rewards and reinforcers to offer to patients, it is crucial to pick something which is important to them (not to us).

UR1, UR2 were excavated and dressed with glass ionomer cement (GIC). This semi-temporary dressing, though far from being a perfect restorative treatment, fulfilled Josh's desire to radically improve his appearance. Such dressings are also quicker and more easily achieved than composite restorations. The vitality of UR2 was tested with a view to long-term monitoring prior to definitive treatment. Josh was delighted with his achievements and the results.

Traditional glass ionomer cements have been used extensively since the 1970s. Glass ionomers have the following properties:
- They self-adhere to enamel and dentine.
- Setting is an acid–base reaction, is water dependent and takes over 24 h for the process to be complete.
- They release fluoride. However, there is no evidence to show a therapeutic benefit associated with fluoride release from this, or any other, dental material.
- They are brittle with low fracture strength and high wear rates when compared with other tooth-coloured restoratives.
- They have poor appearance, especially in respect of opacity, when compared with other tooth-coloured restoratives.
- Stains build up over time.

Glass ionomers are therefore excellent for temporary restorations or as an intermediate restorative to allow stabilization, perhaps in a patient at high caries risk such as Josh. The other situation where glass ionomers are suitable is the restoration of root caries.

3. Third visit: LL1, LR1 were restored with composite under IHS and local anaesthesia.
4. Fourth visit: UL1, UL2 were restored with composite under IHS and local anaesthesia.

Josh was then aged 10. Josh was then given a general anaesthetic appointment for extraction of his first permanent molars. It may have been possible to restore at least some of these teeth, but LR6 required extraction and because of the poor long-term prognosis of the other 6s, it was felt to be in Josh's best interests to remove all four teeth.

If one of the four first permanent molars (FPM) is causing pain and is of poor long-term prognosis, it is important to plan its extraction and, at the same time, consider whether the planned extraction of other first permanent molars might be in the patient's best interests. When a child is in the mixed dentition stage, as Josh is, carefully planned extractions can obviate other problems.

If lower FPMs are to be removed, the optimum time to extract is when calcification of the bifurcation of the second permanent molar has commenced. This is because prior to the development of the bifurcation, when the FPM is removed, the second permanent molar loses the 'prop', which helps to maintain it upright. Thus, if FPMs are removed early, the second molars tend to tip into the FPM space. Combined with distal drift of the second premolar into the FPM space, this can result in a very bad contact between a distally tipped premolar and a mesial tipping molar. Such a contact leads to food trapping and potentially to lack of self-cleansing in the area.

If FPMs are removed late (after the age of 12) residual spacing and rotation of the second premolar can occur.

It is particularly important to consider the state of all four FPMs if the extraction of one is considered. Most especially, this is true in children in whom orthodontic treatment would be contraindicated. Given his extremely high rate of decay and poor oral hygiene, Josh would certainly fit this category.

In Josh's case, one FPM must be extracted and the others had a guarded prognosis. Josh had premolar crowding and it is best to take out both lower FPMs at the time when the bifurcation of the second permanent molars had just formed, thereby relieving the crowding. In Josh's case, the upper FPMs were of doubtful prognosis and were therefore also extracted. In any case, if the lower FPMs are removed, it is usual to extract the upper FPMs to prevent their over-eruption.

Josh's mother and father attended with him for the GA appointment.

Between the visits described above, there were many cancelled and broken appointments. This, the Grandma revealed, was because Josh was so often in youth court. He was playing truant, staying out until after midnight, had been arrested for burning cars and was not attending school.

Despite his very young age Josh appears to have declined into delinquency. Notwithstanding that and the apparent difficulties in providing treatment the dentist should continue to provide care to the best of his/her ability in the circumstances. There would of course be no justification for refusing to treat Josh because of his delinquent tendencies, unless of course the dentist's car was one of the cars that Josh had torched, but the repeated failures to attend may allow the dentist to 'de-register' Josh, thereby relieving him/her of any continuing duty of care.

Three years later: Josh attended again, aged 13, accompanied by his mother. He said that food is getting 'stuck' in his back teeth. When asked if Josh was now attending school, his mother stated that he was not and that he had twice absconded from home and lived rough for five days, one of these occasions being very recent. Josh's mum said that he would eat very little except 'custard cream' biscuits which he ate at the rate of three to four packets per day.

On examination (for which Josh was very cooperative without the need for sedation) the anterior 'semi-permanent' restorations were still in place. Further cavities had developed in LL1, LR1. The second permanent molars were fully erupted, as were the canines and premolars. Visual signs of caries were seen in all four second permanent molars.

Radiographs showed very deep cavities in LR7, LL7 and cavities in UR7, UL7. The oral hygiene was very poor.

Treatment options

1. Extract all second permanent molars under general anaesthetic. Preventive regime, and restorations as required, if attendance permitted. Extract anterior teeth under LA/sedation when there are signs or symptoms.
2. Restore UR7, UL7 under IHS and LA. Extract LL7, LR7 under IHS and LA. Extract anterior teeth when there are signs or symptoms and supply partial denture.
3. Extract all remaining teeth and provide F/F denture.

Once again, Josh had provided a treatment planning dilemma of the most extreme kind. Any faith in his ability to maintain any kind of oral health regime had clearly been misplaced (this was obviously not Josh's fault, more the fault of his circumstances), and yet to remove further problems by providing dentures for a still-growing jaw seemed almost cruel.

Broken, unstable families and family problems often lead to a weakening of parental control over basic food and sleeping habits (which is probably where Josh's problems started). What we also see here is the potential for these problems to proceed in a continuous downward spiral. Research has shown that health-related problems to some extent carry over from one generation to the next and that a process of social reproduction of socioeconomic inequalities in lifestyles can be demonstrated. The theory of learned helplessness discussed earlier is also important here as it helps us to understand how feelings of helplessness and non-control can feed into negative health behaviours and a lack of motivation to engage in behaviours to improve health.

In terms of actual dental health, data have shown that there is a link between lower social class, poverty, and child dental health. Some studies have shown that the social consequences surrounding the environments of poor children, and often the manner in which such children are reared (e.g. the unpredictability associated with parental drug users), are predictive of misbehaviour during dental appointments, especially amongst younger age groups. It is important to realize that the behaviour of such children, just like Josh's behaviour, is a learned response to the environment they are living in. The dentist must try and be sensitive to the problems of such children (and adults) and be prepared to put in extra time and energy that may be needed in dealing with such patients, both before and during dental appointments.

The dentist opted for the first of the treatment plans, i.e. extraction of all second permanent molars under general anaesthetic; however, when this was discussed, Josh asked whether anyone ever died under general anaesthetic. The dentist attempted to describe the probability of such an event using the analogy of one person out of two football stadia full of people. Josh insisted that he might be that one person who was unlucky. In fact, his words were: 'knowing me, I'll be that one'. The dentist could sort of see his point!

Thus, the issue of the personal autonomy of children and consent made it necessary to change the treatment plan to option 2.

It is very important that children are involved in decision-making in respect of treatment which involves them. However, they must be of sufficient maturity to be involved in any discussion between them, their parents, and the dentist, and decisions must be based on the professional advice of the dentist. In the absence of a parent the law determines that a child of sufficient maturity and understanding to make their own mind up on a matter can give legally valid consent (the 'Gillick competent child'). Evidence of a lack of maturity may be taken where the child takes a decision to refuse treatment which is clearly in their best interests, and based upon misconceptions or misunderstanding of the risks involved. Clearly the greater the threat to their well-being then the greater the maturity required.

Even with a Gillick competent child, consent, or refusal, is not valid if the information upon which it is based is not adequate. Here Josh has based his decision upon the fact that one person out of two full football stadia die under general anaesthesia. What is the ratio? How big is each stadium? Is that true? Is that all general anaesthetics given or just those for dental treatment? Does it include those deaths arising from gross negligence, of which there have been many in the past decade, or just the inherent risk? Is it the best way to present such risks in any event? Josh is clearly influenced, however, by this 'statistic' and it illustrates the importance of giving adequate information in an appropriate manner.

Involving children, either Gillick competent or not, in the decision-making process does not present any problems when they agree with dentist, and/or their parents. If Josh's mother wished him to have general anaesthesia and it was really the only option available for the extraction of four painful and infected molar teeth, if he is not considered to be Gillick competent there is not a problem, as consent can come from one of the parents, or whoever has parental responsibility. If Josh is considered Gillick competent this illustrates the delicate moral balance between autonomy and the obligation of beneficence—the duty to do good for the patient. In the case of an adult, as you are aware, it is not a problem. In the case of a child the difficulty is that respecting the child's self-determination runs counter to the dentist's and the parents' duty and desire to care for the child and stop the pain. Morally it is a fine balance. Legally too. There is clear legal authority stating that the consent of the parent would be legally valid up to the age of 18 years. The legal power to overrule the child in such circumstances is given on the basis of the welfare, both physical and psychological, of the child being of paramount importance. It is to be exercised after very careful consideration. There is no guidance, but it is suggested that it should be restricted to occasions where the chid is a risk of serious and/or irreversible harm.

At the next visit, at which UR7, UL7 were to be restored under LA and sedation, Josh was accompanied by his aunt. She explained that he was now living with her and was attending a new school, which catered particularly for boys with Josh's kinds of difficulties. She was very concerned about the need for extractions of permanent teeth and stated that it was her and Josh's wish that he kept his teeth if at all possible. The very poor state of, and prognosis for, the teeth were explained. Also Josh was anxious about the extractions. Given that the treatment plan was far from ideal, the dentist agreed to investigate the teeth and restore them if at all possible.

When Josh attends for treatment under sedation, he is accompanied by his aunt, whom the dentist has not met before, and with whom Josh is now living. The dentist is unaware of the basis of that arrangement. There are once again consent issues here. However, on the basis of previous discussions involving Josh and his mother regarding treatment and Josh's refusal of general anaesthesia, Josh appears to be Gillick competent for the sedation and the treatment being provided. It would seem, however, that restoration of the second molars is a treatment option that the dentist considers second best, that their extraction is treatment of choice. This raises an ethical problem. Once again it illustrates the conflict between autonomy and beneficence. If one further considers the moral obligation of non-maleficence (to do no harm) then the problem is more easily resolved. The balance of beneficence and non-maleficence represents the best interests of the patient. The patient is in reality the only person who can determine their best interests based upon information provided by the dentist. In attempting to restore Josh's teeth the harm that may result is that the treatment may fail. He may suffer further pain in the future. The teeth may need to be extracted at a later date. This does not constitute harm as the dentist would like to extract them now. If Josh, and/or his mother, or whoever may be required to consent on his behalf, are fully informed, then both morally and legally there are no difficulties in following this second treatment option, provided that it is clinically reasonable and not obviously against the patient's best interests.

On examining Josh's mouth, the dentist noted that it was considerably cleaner. The aunt said that now that Josh had a more settled life, he would be taking better care of his mouth and that his diet was now much better.

The dentist then proceeded to open the UL7, which required antibiotic steroid dressing as it was cariously exposed.

Ledermix is a proprietary paste containing a tetracycline antibiotic (demeclocycline) as its antibacterial agent and a corticosteroid (triamcinolone) as an anti-inflammatory agent. The release of demeclocycline is short-lived and it has a limited spectrum of antibiotic action. If an antibacterial action is the desired goal then other agents, such as zinc oxide eugenol, are more effective since eugenol has a broader spectrum of antibacterial action and its release is much more sustained. However, the triamcinolone component makes Ledermix a very effective short-term pulp sedative. Triamcinolone is released rapidly, moving through dentine to the pulp in a few hours. Sixty per cent of the available steroid is released during the first day and virtually all is gone by 2 to 3 days. Ledermix has a palliative effect on the pulp for a short period of time. In a healthy pulp, reparative dentine will continue to be formed between the Ledermix and the pulp.

The dilemma regarding extraction thus remained.

Josh was not seen again until years later.

Six years later, aged 19, Josh attended with severe pain in the lower left quadrant. The anterior teeth all had large open cavities. Josh looked thin and unwell.

On questioning, he admitted that he had been a heroin addict from aged 16. Recently (in the past 6 months) he had been treated with methadone in an attempt to break his habit.

Methadone is an opioid substitute used as part of the treatment of dependence on opioid drugs. The possible benefits of methadone programmes include reductions in levels of needle use, illicit drug use, and criminal activity and improvement in individual lifestyles.

Methadone is usually taken orally as a viscous sugary syrup and is rapidly absorbed from the gastrointestinal tract. This obviates the need for the use of needles, and as it has a long half-life this may help prevent symptoms of withdrawal. The frequent intake and prolonged retention of methadone syrup may result in high levels of dental caries. Sorbitol is being substituted for sucrose as well as methylcellulose or gum tragacanth to render the preparation less cariogenic and more difficult to inject. Although a sugar-free version is available and may reduce the cariogenicity of methadone, other aspects of drug-users' lifestyles may result in high caries levels. General, personal neglect and a shortage of money may lead an opioid user to have a diet based on cheap easily accessible ready-to-eat foods which are high in refined carbohydrates. It is thought that opioids can directly induce a craving for sweet carbohydrates and can also result in xerostomia. Both of these factors may contribute to increased caries levels often seen in addicts.

Josh tells the dentist that he has his own house which he shares with his 17-year-old girlfriend and his 1-year-old son, whom he clearly adores. He was concerned about the rapidly deteriorating appearance of his mouth and of course the almost intolerable pain he was suffering.

When a medical history was taken, Josh said that he had been seriously ill with liver disease. He had been told this was due to using dirty needles to inject. He was also HIV positive.

Medical histories should cover:
- Anything that might result in an emergency, e.g. epilepsy, allergies, diabetes.
- If modifications need to be made to the dental treatment that can be provided, or to the matter in which treatment is delivered, e.g. latex allergy.
- Whether the patient may need medical care prior to dental care, e.g. susceptibility to infective endocarditis, bleeding tendencies.
- If the patient may be a risk to other patients or staff, e.g. through infections, violence, or intoxication.

Some patients resent being questioned about their medical history, especially in the case of transmissible diseases and/or drug abuse. HIV infection is a particularly delicate matter as a patient may be offended by direct questioning. Opioid drugs may alter behaviour and have a potential for interacting with drugs used in dental care. For these reasons, it is important to try and get the patient to reveal all the relevant details of their medical history.

However, there is no guarantee that any of the answers given are honest and the policy should be to treat all patients in a similar manner regarding infection control.

Treatment of high-risk patients

Health-care workers are often reluctant to deal with these patients, yet there are increasing numbers of patients with HIV, hepatitis B, C or D infections. Reluctance may relate to concerns about cross-infection, distrust of abusers' motives for seeking care, concern about inconsistent behaviour, or how other patients in the practice may feel about such patients. Identification of high-risk patients may be difficult, especially in drug addicts. Signs to look for include abnormal behaviour, persistently constricted pupils, and outlining of veins.

Along with the increased probability of a drug addict being the carrier of a blood-borne virus, the potential difficulties in providing dental treatment for drug addicts include:

- providing analgesia,
- behavioural disturbances,
- poor attendance patterns,
- feigning of pain in order to acquire analgesics,
- theft of prescription forms or drugs.

Blood-borne viruses

Dentists will inevitably come into contact with blood and saliva and may be exposed to pathogens including blood-borne viruses such as HIV and hepatitis B and C. It is impossible to identify all patients with infection, blood-borne or otherwise. It is recommended that all body fluids are regarded as potentially infectious and universal precautions be used.

The most common means of transmission is direct contact, particularly via hands. Blood-borne infections are most likely to be transmitted by direct per-cutaneous inoculation of infected blood via a sharps injury. Risks of trans-mission following a needlestick injury are:

- hepatitis B 30%,
- hepatitis C 3%,
- HIV 0.3%.

Universal precautions against infection

- Hand washing or the use of alcoholic hand rubs (when hands have not been physically dirtied).
- Cuts and abrasions in any area of exposed skin should be covered with a dressing, which is waterproof, breathable, and is an effective viral and bacterial barrier.
- Seamless, non-powdered gloves should be worn whenever contact with body fluids is anticipated. Sterile gloves are required for invasive pro-cedures.
- Visors, goggles, or safety spectacles should be worn whenever splashing with body fluids or flying contaminated debris/tissue is anticipated.
- Water-repellent masks to be worn when there is a risk of blood splash to the face.
- Take care during the use and disposal of sharps. Do not re-sheath sharps. Dispose of all sharps at the point of use into an approved sharps container.
- All waste contaminated with blood or body fluids must be discarded into clinical waste sacks, labelled, and sent for incineration according to local policy.
- All health-care workers who perform exposure-prone procedures must be immunized against hepatitis B.

- The patient's medical history should be checked at every visit and updated yearly.
- Work surfaces should be cleaned with detergent, dried, then wiped with 70% isopropyl alcohol.
- Instruments and equipment should be cleaned (in a washer disinfector, ultrasonic bath, or manually in a sink), rinsed, and dried before autoclaving.
- Vacuum extraction autoclaves are the best method of sterilizing dental instruments, principally due to the fine lumen in handpieces and suction equipment.

Significant injury or exposure

'Significant' injuries are defined as exposure to blood or other high-risk body fluid through:
- skin puncture by a sharp object,
- splashing of broken skin,
- splashing of eyes or mouth.

General first aid procedures in the event of all 'significant' injuries or exposures

- Puncture wounds: Encourage bleeding from the puncture site. Do not suck. Wash the area thoroughly with soap and water. Cover with a waterproof dressing.
- Splashes to mucous membranes: Irrigate with copious amounts of sterile water.

Reducing the risk of hepatitis B after 'significant' exposure to high-risk body fluids

In addition to general first aid measures you may need hepatitis B immunoglobulin (HBIG) and/or hepatitis B vaccine after a 'significant' injury in order to reduce your risk of becoming infected with hepatitis B.

Reducing the risk of HIV after 'significant' exposure to high-risk body fluids

In addition to general first aid measures, starting treatment with post-exposure prophylaxis (PEP) is recommended with oral antiviral chemotherapy to reduce the risk of HIV transmission if you have had a 'significant' exposure to blood or other high-risk body fluids from an identifiable patient (the 'source') and the source is known or strongly suspected to be in one of the following groups:
- HIV antibody positive,
- an injecting drug user,
- a gay/bisexual man,
- a sex industry worker,
- from an area endemic for HIV, for example sub-Saharan Africa.

    In the case of 'significant' exposure to high-risk body fluids from a source not in any of the above high-risk groups, or from an unknown source, the risk of HIV infection is too small to justify PEP because of the side-effects from treatment.

After taking a careful medical history from Josh, an intra-oral radiographic examination revealed the following:
1. Gross caries of all remaining teeth.
2. Pulpal involvement of badly broken down upper incisors, second permanent molars and lower centrals.
3. Periapical pathology of LR7.
4. Draining sinuses UR2, UL1.
5. 'High-risk' patient.

   The prognosis for the remaining teeth is extremely poor. The chance of Josh attending regularly for root treatments/crowns was, in the dentist's view, zero, even if this were a viable treatment option. Doing nothing was also not an option due to Josh's severe pain.

Because Josh is clearly in severe pain, morally, doing nothing is not an option. The dentist must attempt to relieve and/or make appropriate arrangements for immediate pain relief. The fact of Josh's HIV status is not an issue as to the provision of treatment. If the dentist is able to provide treatment and effect pain relief then s/he ought to do so. The General Dental Council is clear in its view on the treatment of patients with HIV. This moral obligation is not supported by the law at present. The dentist would only be justified in referring Josh for this treatment if there was a clinical basis for the referral.

Thus, this seemed to be one of those extremely rare cases whereby clearance of the remaining teeth and provision of a denture appeared to be the only sensible option.

When Josh was 13, the dentist was persuaded by Josh's aunt, and his apparently happier and healthier potential future, to avoid extractions of the upper molars, though they had an extremely poor prognosis even at that stage. By attempting 'heroics' in such a disease-prone mouth and in such a spasmodically attending patient the dentist was committing a patient to a lifetime of repair and restoration which he was very unlikely to maintain, let alone afford. The opportunity to remove the teeth was lost once the patient's pain was resolved by utilizing medicaments in the tooth.

   Given the way events transpired for Josh, it is arguable that the wrong decision was made when he was 13. However, removal of the only remaining molar teeth in a 13-year-old is a very hard action to justify. Josh of course represents an extreme case but such cases do exist and can offer dentists some of their most difficult treatment decision-making dilemmas.

BIBLIOGRAPHY

Abramson L, Seligman M, Teasdale J. Learned helplessness in humans: critique and reformulation. *Journal of Abnormal Psychology* 1978; **87**: 49–74.

Arseneault L, Tremblay R, Boulerice B, Seguin J, Saucier J. Minor physical anomalies and family adversity as risk factors for violent delinquency in adolescence. *American Journal of Psychiatry* 2000; **157**(6): 917–923.

Attkisson C, Zich J (eds). *Depression in Primary Care: Screening and Detection*. Routledge: London, 1990.

Bandolier Extra: Evidence-based Healthcare. *Needlesticks*, July 2003. www.jr2.ox.ac.uk/bandolier/Extraforbando/needle.pdf

Blinkhorn AS, Mackie IC. *Practical Treatment Planning for the Paediatric Patient*. Quintessence: London, 1992.

Bridgman CM, Ashley D, Holloway PJ. An investigation of the effects on children of tooth extraction under general anaesthesia. *British Dental Journal* 1999; **186**: 245–247.

Brunton PA. *Decision Making in Operative Dentistry*. Quintessence: London, 2002.

Chaiken S. Communicator physical attractiveness and persuasion. *Journal of Personal and Social Psychology* 1979; **37**: 1387–1397.

Cohen LK, Gift HC (eds). *Disease Prevention and Oral Health Promotion. Socio-dental Sciences in Action*. Munksgaard: Copenhagen, 1995.

Crossley ML, Joshi G. An investigation of paediatric dentists' attitudes towards parental accompaniment and behavioural techniques in the UK. *British Dental Journal* 2002; **192**: 517–521.

DiBase A, Sandler P. Malocclusion, orthodontics and bullying. *Dental Update* 2001; **28**(9): 646–9.

Downs A, Lyons P. Natural observations of the links between attractiveness and initial legal judgements. *Journal of Personal and Social Psychology Bulletin* 1995; **17**: 541–547.

Fayle SA, Wellbury RR, Roberts JF. British Society of Paediatric Dentistry. A policy document on management of caries in the primary dentition. *International Journal of Paediatric Dentistry* 2001; **11**: 153–157.

Gillick v West Norfolk and Wisbech Area Health Authority [1985] 3 All ER 402.

Hammermesh D, Biddle J. Beauty and the labour market. *American Economic Review* 1994; **84**: 1174–1195.

Hinds K, Gregory JK. *National Diet and Nutrition Survey: Children Aged $1\frac{1}{2}$ to $4\frac{1}{2}$ Years. Vol 2. Report of the Dental Survey*. HMSO: London, 1995.

Jacob MC, Plamping D. *The Practice of Primary Dental Care*. Wright: London, 1989.

Kay EJ. The psychology of behaviour change and dental health. *Dental Update* 1988; **15**: 386–389.

Kay EJ, Locker D. *Effectiveness of Oral Health Promotion: A Review*. HEA: London, 1997.

Kay EJ, Nuttall NM. *Clinical Decision Making. An Art or a Science?* BDJ Books: London, 1997.

Kay EJ, Tinsley S. Children—special cases. *Communication for the Dental Team*, ch.8. Partners in Practice: Northants, 1995.

Ketterlinus R, Lamb M, Nitz K. Adolescent non-sexual and sex related problem behaviours. Their prevalence, consequences and co-occurrence. In: Ketterlinus R and Lamb M (eds). *Adolescent Problem Behaviours. Issues and Research*. Erlbaum Associates: Mahwah, NJ, 1994.

Killen M, Crystal D, Watanabe H. Japanese and American children's evaluations of peer exclusion, tolerance of differences, and prescriptions for conformity. *Child Development* 2002; **73**(6): 1788–1802.

Langlois J, Roggman L, Musselman L. What is average and what is not average about attractive faces? *Psychological Science* 1994; **5**: 214–220.

Muir Gray JA. *The Resourceful Patient*. Rossetta Press: Oxford, 2002.

Pierson C. Effects of virtual baldness intervention on the peer popularity ratings of children. *Dissertation Abstracts International. Section B: the Sciences and Engineering* 2001; **61**(9-B): 4967. (University Microfilms International.)

Pine CM, McGoldrick PM, Burnside G, Curnow MH, Chesters RK, Nicolson J, Huntington E. An intervention programme to establish regular toothbrushing: understanding parents beliefs and motivating children. *International Dental Journal* 2000; **50**: 312–323.

Pinkham J, Casamassimo P, Levy S. Dentistry and the children of poverty. *Journal of Dentistry for Children* 1988; **55**(1): 17–24.

Pitts NB, Evans DJ, Nugent ZJ. The dental caries of 5 year old children in Great Britain in 1999/2000. Surveys coordinated by the British Association for the Study of Community Dentistry. *Community Dental Health* 2001; **18**: 49–55.

Re J (A Minor) (Medical Treatment) [1992] 3 WLR 758, 3 Med LR 317.

Re R (A Minor) (Wardship: Consent to Treatment) [1992] Fam 11, 3 Med LR 342.

Rotter J. *The Development and Applications of Social Learning Theory: Selected Papers*. Praeger: Brattleboro, VT, 1982.

Tickle M, Williams MJ, Jenner AM, Blinkhorn A. The effects of dental attendance and socio-economic status on dental caries experience and treatment patterns in 5 year old children. *British Dental Journal* 1999; **186**: 135–137.

Titsas A, Ferguson MM. Impact of opioid use on dentistry. *Australian Dental Journal* 2002; **47**(2): 94–98.

Townsend P, Philimore P, Beattie A. *Health and Deprivation: Inequalities in Health*. Croom Helm: London, 1988.

Trzepacz A. Peer acceptance and self-perceptions in children: the impact of gender and race. *Dissertation Abstracts International. Section B: the Sciences and Engineering* 2001; **62**(5-B): 2505. (University Microfilms International.)

Watt R, Sheiham A. Inequalities in oral health: a review of the evidence and recommendations for action. *British Dental Journal* 1999; **187**: 6–7.

Zebrowitz L. McDonald S. The impact of litigants' baby-facedness and attractiveness on adjudications in small claims courts. *Law and Human Behavior* 1991; **15**: 603–623.

David: a law-abiding customer

David is a 28-year-old ex-public schoolboy. He works as a lawyer and plays rugby at district level. He is fit and well (other than hay fever in the summer) and owns his own home, which he shares with his 23-year-old girlfriend who is studying medicine.

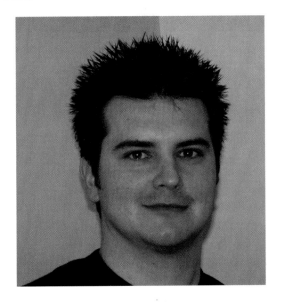

David

Does social background or social class have a direct effect on dental health?

David presents at a dentist's surgery, expressing concerns about the appearance of the crown on UL1. He does not like the dark line which is visible adjacent to his gum and says that the colour of the crown is wrong.

On examination, UL6, UL7 and LL6 are missing. UR6, LR6 and LL6 have full gold crowns and UL1 has a metal ceramic crown. Radiographs show that UR6 and UL1 are root filled. The UL1 crown is indeed a shade lighter than the other crowned teeth but in the dentist's view is not particularly aesthetically unpleasing. The dentist told David this, but he was insistent that he wanted a new crown and said that he was happy to pay privately if that was what was required in order to get the treatment he wanted. The radiographs of the tooth showed that it was restored with a long, parallel-sided post and that the

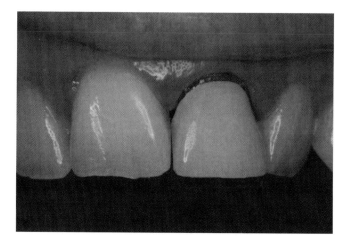

Crown on UL1, with dark gingival margin

remaining root filling material was short of the apex and under-condensed. There was a periradicular radiolucency around the tooth but, as the post and crown had been placed only 6 months ago, it was unclear whether or not the area was healing. The dentist suspected that it was not, as the small amount of root filling material discernible on the radiograph could not possibly have provided an adequate seal, especially in a tooth restored with a post.

Are root treatments an appropriate and evidence-based means of treating non-vital teeth?

Diagnosis

David thus presented with a perceived need for treatment on aesthetic grounds. Although the aesthetic appearance of UL1 was not as good as it might have been, it would have been deemed acceptable by most patients and most dentists. However, there was a potential pathology at the apex of the tooth and a completely inadequate root filling which was unlikely to help resolution of the periapical problem. David was unaware of the inadequacy of the treatment because he was not experiencing any symptoms whatever from the tooth. Removal of the current crown and replacement of the root filling might therefore create problems for David which did not currently exist. There was also concern about what David's reaction would be if he was informed that the previous treatment was inadequate, quite apart from the aesthetic aspects.

What should the dentist tell David?

Should he replace the crown, and what should he do about the apparently inadequate root canal treatment?

Treatment options

1. The dentist could refuse to give David any active treatment at present but suggest that he returns in 6 months for a further periapical radiograph of the tooth so that he can assess whether bony infill is occurring.

2. The dentist could replace the crown and leave the post and root fillings *in situ*, then monitor as per option 1.
3. The dentist could attempt to remove the post, root fill the tooth again, then make a new post and crown.
4. The dentist could carry out periradicular surgery, wait for it to settle, then, if successful, replace the crown.

All of these options have advantages and disadvantages. These must be conveyed to the patient.

Which of the treatment options above would you choose, and why?

Unfortunately, despite it being important to discuss the pros and cons of treatment, after discussing the issues David said he wished to sue his previous dentist for not treating him properly. David then said that, out of the options the dentist had offered, he wanted the crown to be replaced.

What should you do about David's threat to sue the previous dentist?
What prompts patients to complain and sue when an adverse outcome occurs?

The dentist accepted David's wishes and undertook the treatment, making careful notes. Eighteen months later, David attended the practice for a check-up. The dentist was unable to detect any changes in the quality of the bone surrounding the apex of UL1. It was no better but had not got any worse.

David plays rugby at quite a high level, so at each visit the dentist adjured him to wear the mouth guard he had made for him. David admits that he does not always do so as, he says, he cannot breathe well with it in, and the 'lads' cannot understand what he shouts to them when there is a lineout. The dentist feels obliged to warn him that he has very expensive dentistry in his mouth and that a blow to a post crown would undoubtedly cause loss of the tooth.

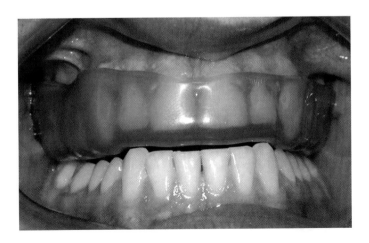

A well-fitting mouthguard

Is the threat of 'poor' outcomes sufficient to motivate patients?

A week and a half later, David attends the surgery again. He is off-colour and in incredible pain from UL1. He said that he wore his mouth guard at his last rugby match but had been punched in the face at least twice during the game. David could not bear UL1 even to be touched and he said that he has been unable to either eat or sleep since Sunday night (3 days ago).

Aggressively, David demands that the dentist get him out of pain. The dentist explained that it would be difficult to achieve adequate anaesthesia for extracting the tooth or in order to undertake any other type of treatment.

David begs again for the dentist to do something and yet he cannot bear have the tooth or surrounding mucosa touched. A radiograph (taken with difficulty) showed pretty much the same appearance as the previous two, which were taken at David's check-ups. The dentist feels under terrible pressure to take the tooth out, as David is so upset, and is desperate for the source of the pain to be removed.

What would you do under these circumstances?
What are the treatment options, which would you choose, and why?

After much discussion about the options, David agrees that, although he desperately wishes to be out of pain and wants the tooth removed, he would have the crown removed and keep the tooth root.

What anaesthetic technique would be appropriate in this case?

Using an appropriate anaesthetic technique the crown was removed by cutting it off with a burr. The post was then removed using an ultrasonic tip and drainage through the tooth achieved, giving David substantial relief from his pain. Once the acute infection subsided, a well-condensed root filling was placed in the apical third of the root and a post core and crown provided. The

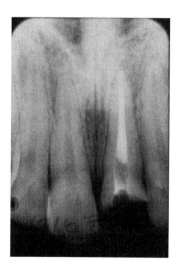

Radiograph showing well condensed root filling in UL1

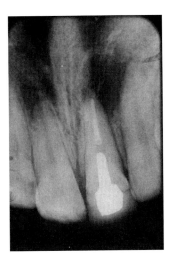

Radiograph showing periradicular
radiolucency in UL1, now restored with
post-retained crown

shade was carefully chosen in consultation with David and he appeared to be
very happy with the result. However, 12 months later, David presented again
with pain from the same tooth.

On radiographing the tooth, although the root filling looked extremely good,
a well-defined radiolucency, approximately 0.75 cm in diameter, with a rim of
well condensed bone, was visible. This was diagnosed as a cyst. The only sensible option at this stage was to perform periradicular surgery.

What are the clinical indications for apicecting a tooth?

Would you be liable if you undertook an apicectomy and it failed?

David asked whether the periradicular surgery procedure would give him a
really good chance of keeping his tooth and the dentist said that it would.

What is the success rate of periradicular surgery?

The periradicular surgery was duly performed and the cyst curetted out. On
inspection, during the periradicular surgery, the seal at the root face appeared
to be sound so no retrograde root filling was placed.

What is the procedure for apicectomy?

The healing after the procedure was uneventful. However, 3 weeks and two
courses of antibiotics later, David was still experiencing symptoms from the
tooth.

The treatment options at this stage were:

1. Repeat the surgery on the tooth.
2. Extract the tooth and replace with: an implant; a conventional bridge; a
   resin retained bridge; a cobalt-chrome denture; or nothing.

Option 1 is a possibility but the chances of success diminish each time a
tooth is apicectomized. Given that David had hoped for a positive outcome from
the first procedure and had then experienced a negative one, it is unlikely that

he would, if given this information, wish to proceed. Indeed, when the odds of success are explained to David, he becomes angry and seeks a second opinion, saying he will sue if he has been 'messed up'.

How can you manage a patient who starts to show anger?

However, having visited two further dentists, who offered him similar treatment, David returns to your surgery, apologizing for his behaviour and anger, and asks whether you would remove the tooth and place an implant.

Was it acceptable for David to ask other dentists' opinions?
Do you have to undertake David's continued treatment?

The dentist agrees to undertake the treatment and, after a long discussion with David about the pros and cons of such treatment, places a single tooth implant.

What is the likelihood that the implant will be successful?

For several years after the fitting of the single tooth implant, David attends regularly for check-ups and treatment when required. He has one or two pieces of conventional restorative work done but nothing major. David then stops attending and nothing is heard of him for 4 years.

The dentist then received a letter from a casualty department:

Dear

Mr David Lester has been attending this casualty department for treatment of a broken left mandible which he sustained in a fight in Anytown Rugby Club. The police were involved and legal action may result from their enquiries.

In the meantime, whilst David was under our treatment for the fracture, it was noted that he required some routine dental treatment. He gave your name as his dentist and we are therefore writing so that you are aware of the fracture which was treated using two finger plates and of the circumstances in which the injuries were sustained.

Yours sincerely

Several days later, David rings for a dental appointment. When he attends, he complains of pain in the joint of his jaw on the right-hand side. He also needs two restorations. These are carried out but David continues to complain about the pain in his 'jaw joint'. His occlusion seems no different from previously and no signs of temporomandibular joint (TMJ) disease (pain, click, muscle tenderness, deviation) can be detected.

David says that the pain is so bad that he cannot work. He asks the dentist if he will come to court and say that the pain was due to the injuries he sustained in the fight.

Does David have TMJ problems?
Will the court ask you to appear?

DAVID: A LAW-ABIDING CITIZEN

David is a 28-year-old ex-public schoolboy. He works as a lawyer and plays rugby at district level. He is fit and well (other than hay fever in the summer) and owns his own home, which he shares with his 23-year-old girlfriend who is studying medicine.

There are marked social inequalities in child health across the UK. For example there is a six-fold difference in the amount of dental decay in 5-year-old children in Glasgow (inner city) when compared with Solihull (affluent area). Of interest is whether inequalities in children are reflected in the oral health of adults and adolescents. Inequalities may be due to parental upbringing, school environment, earlier access to dental checks, and more frequent asymptomatic visits. It is known that registration is higher in higher social groups (81%) than in lower social groups (67%). Most industrialized countries demonstrate a socioeconomic gradient in the adoption of dental services. People with low income and less education tend to show poorer health, possibly because of poorer attendance at the dentist but possibly also because of lower take-up of preventive services. Diet regimes and general health and hygiene behaviours at school and at home are likely to be more dentally healthy in high-income households.

David presents at a dentist's surgery expressing concerns about the appearance of the crown on UL1. He does not like the dark line which is visible adjacent to his gum and says that the colour of the crown is wrong.

On examination, UL6, UL7 and LL6 are missing. UR6, LR6 and LL6 have full gold crowns and UL1 has a metal ceramic crown. Radiographs show that UR6 and UL1 are root filled. The UL2 crown is indeed a shade lighter than the other crowned teeth but in the dentist's view is not particularly aesthetically unpleasing. The dentist told David this, but he was insistent that he wanted a new crown and said that he was happy to pay privately if that was what was required in order to get the treatment he wanted. The radiographs of the tooth showed that it was restored with a long, parallel-sided post and that the remaining root filling material was short of the apex and under-condensed. There was a periradicular radiolucency around the tooth but, as the post and crown had been placed only 6 months ago, it was unclear whether or not the area was healing. The dentist suspected that it was not, as the small amount of root filling material discernible on the radiograph could not possibly have provided an adequate seal, especially in a tooth restored with a post.

Root treatment

The aim of root treatment is to eliminate the bacteria (the origin of the pulpal/periradicular disease) from the root canal system and seal the canal space to prevent bacteria re-entering the canal spaces. Canals are prepared to remove any remaining pulp tissue, bacteria, and irritants from the canal and to provide a tapered canal preparation. This is usually carried out using hand files or rotary instruments in conjunction with an irrigant, such as sodium hypochlorite. To obtain a seal the canal spaces are obturated, normally with gutta percha and a sealer, then a coronal seal of glass ionomer or bonding resin is placed over the gutta percha. Ideally the root canal filling should be well condensed to within 1 mm of the radiographic apex. However, it should be remembered that a number of factors affect the outcome of root canal treatment, including the quality of the root filling, isolation, the use of disinfecting medicaments, and the presence of a coronal seal.

Root canal treatment is 83–94% successful in well-controlled studies, however, in epidemiological studies the success rate is 61–77%. Published studies have shown that only 30–40% of root fillings would be rated as acceptable according to the criteria laid down by various authorities (i.e. radiographically dense and 0–2 mm from the radiographic apex). The quality of the root filling is therefore not the only factor affecting outcome. The quality of the coronal seal has a significant impact on the success of root canal treatment.

Diagnosis

David thus presented with a perceived need for treatment on aesthetic grounds. Although the aesthetic appearance of UL1 was not as good as it might have been, it would have been deemed acceptable by most patients and most dentists. However, there was a potential pathology at the apex of the tooth and a completely inadequate root filling which was unlikely to help resolution of the periapical problem. David was unaware of the inadequacy of the treatment because he was not experiencing any symptoms whatever from the tooth. Removal of the current crown and replacement of the root filling might therefore create problems for David which did not currently exist. There was also concern about what David's reaction would be if he was informed that the previous treatment was inadequate, quite apart from the aesthetic aspects.

David has presented requesting aesthetic improvement of the crown at UL1, which was placed just 6 months previously. It is important to find out why David has not returned to the dentist who placed it. That in itself ought to alert any dentist to the possibility of difficulties ahead. Maybe David fell out with the previous dentist or maybe his request for treatment was refused for some reason. The tooth has a dark line at gingival level of UL1 and it is a shade lighter than the crowns on his other front teeth, but the dentist does not consider that the appearance of the crown to be aesthetically displeasing. He would, however, seem to think that although the appearance was not as good as it could have been, it would be accepted by most patients. Of course, the crown must be an adequate fit, otherwise there would be no debate about whether it needed to be replaced. There is a clinical issue, because although the UL1 was root treated 6 months ago, the root canal filling is completely inadequate.

The first question to be addressed is the inadequate root canal filling. While it is not known whether the periapical radiolucency is healing or not, the root canal filling does not provide an adequate apical seal. David should be advised of this. It would be important to try to obtain a more detailed history in respect of the crowned upper incisors, particularly, if possible, the reason for root canal treatment at UL1. Following that, future treatment options can be fully discussed. The dentist must be careful to avoid any criticism of the previous dentist's treatment. There may be a number of reasons for the poor quality of the root canal filling, which may not necessarily mean that the previous dentist has been negligent. However, upon completion and prior to the placement of the post crown, the previous dentist should have known of the poor quality root filling and advised David accordingly. In the absence of any symptoms the best treatment option might be to leave the post in place, in view of the risks inherent in its removal. The tooth could then be kept under review. Although this is a clinical decision, it is one which must be reached in consultation with David.

If there is clinical need to replace the crown, or if it is to be replaced in accordance with David's request, then David ought to be advised of his need to have the root filling replaced. If not, then it is possible that within a very short time of the new crown being fitted David will suffer from an acute flare-up at UL1.

It would appear that there is no dental clinical need to replace the crown, although the dark line at the gingival margin is undoubtedly unaesthetic. The problem is that there is a difference of opinion between David and the dentist in the perceived aesthetic quality of the crown. The issue here is whose view should prevail. This raises the question of acting in the patient's best interests, the principle of beneficence—doing what is 'best'—which, in interventional health care, is usually a net balance of doing good and not doing harm. It is a matter that defers to autonomy. Both the patient and the dentist have personal autonomy. All the risks of replacing the crown should be explained to David. The benefits are obvious to him. David will then be in a position to decide whether or not replacement of the crown will be in his best interests. He alone knows the true effect that the slight aesthetic problem has upon his sense of well-being. He is the only one who can truly weigh up the risks against the hoped for aesthetic improvement. There could be no criticism of the dentist for acceding to David's request so long as this conversation had taken place and David felt that there was a benefit to be gained by having the crown replaced.

However, the dentist too has autonomy. If the dentist believes that replacement is not necessary, i.e. s/he cannot see or agree with David's perceived need, then s/he is not compelled to replace the crown as requested, although the dentist would be no doubt criticized for taking such a stance. In such circumstances, the dentist ought to set out her/his reasons to David and explain that other dentists may take a different approach to the request and that he ought to seek a further opinion.

Treatment options

1. The dentist could refuse to give David any active treatment at present but suggest that he returns in 6 months for a further periapical radiograph of the tooth so that he can assess whether bony infill is occurring.

2. The dentist could replace the crown and leave the post and root fillings *in situ*, then monitor as per option 1.
3. The dentist could attempt to remove the post, root fill the tooth again, then make a new post and crown.
4. The dentist could carry out periradicular surgery, wait for it to settle, then, if successful, replace the crown.

All of these options have advantages and disadvantages. These must be conveyed to the patient.

Option 1 is a good one, in as much as the success or otherwise of the current root filling should be established before recrowning the tooth. However, David was obviously very concerned about its appearance and if you refused to give him the treatment he wanted, he would be likely to go and find another dentist who would.

The second option has the advantage of providing David with what he wanted, without involving him in difficult or time-consuming treatments. However, the crown removal may precipitate a flare-up of the periradicular periodontitis. If you were to replace the crown and the periapical situation subsequently deteriorated and caused David pain, you would then have to carry out periradicular surgery, or you would have to remove the post and crown and re-root treat the tooth.

Removing post and crown, as per option 3, enables you to attempt a satisfactory root canal treatment. If this works then a good treatment outcome would be achieved. However, post removal carries with it a degree of risk, particularly in this case where there is a long, parallel-sided post. This post design is very retentive so risk of root fracture is fairly high. Posts may be removed by a number of different methods: either pulled out, trephined out using instruments such as the Masserann kit or more conservatively, removed by use of fine ultrasonic tips. If root fracture does occur, there would be no alternative other than extraction and prosthetic replacement of the tooth.

The last option, of undertaking periradicular surgery would be an excellent one if the patient had had symptoms. It would also be a good option if the probability of success were very high. However, most authorities would agree that periradicular surgery should not be attempted until an adequate root filling has failed to obviate symptoms.

Unfortunately, despite it being important to discuss the pros and cons of treatment, after discussing the issues David said he wished to sue his previous dentist for not treating him properly. David then said that, out of the options the dentist had offered, he wanted the crown to be replaced.

Despite the fact that you were very careful not to criticise the previous dentist about the poor root canal treatment, David has interpreted the existence of a poor quality root canal filling as being due to poor workmanship. In truth he is probably right. In consequence, if the root canal treatment is to be redone, a new post crown will also be required. Clearly David now needs treatment that he would not have required if the root canal treatment had been of a satisfactory standard. Faced with such a situation, the keeping of precise records of the clinical and radiographic findings and of the discussion cannot be more strongly stressed. Should David proceed with his action against the previous dentist you will be requested by David's solicitors to disclose those records and radiographs, unless of course he chooses to represent himself. Any such letter requesting the records ought to have attached a medical records release consent form signed by David. You should never release records, or copies of them, unless such a consent form is received. In these circumstances, it would be prudent to contact your indemnifiers.

Typically, there are at least four triggers for initiating litigation or making a formal complaint. They include:

- The altruistic desire to prevent other patients suffering from similar harm.
- The seriousness of the adverse outcome.
- Being misled and a sense of an individual or individuals attempting to avoid detection.
- Discussion of events informally with others.

For a complaint to develop into a formal proceeding there is nearly always an issue of poor-quality communication. It is important therefore for dentists to observe certain strategies to prevent further action by the offended party. They include the following:

- Dentists should present the possible complications and risks of treatments and interventions that are being considered. Alternative approaches should be related and costs discussed. The length of the treatment, frequency of attendance, and number of procedures and investigations are all aspects that need to be covered.
- Sensitive, open communication should be maintained throughout the episode of care, especially when outcomes are not favourable or known complications arise. This will prevent the patient feeling that they are being ignored. Hence, when things go wrong, an acknowledgement of what has happened is highly desirable.
- Decisions, observations, and discussions with patients should be documented in the written notes to ensure that these details are remembered and the patient knows that you have appreciated and are clearly aware of the issues pertinent to their received treatment and continued care.

The dentist accepted David's wishes and undertook the treatment, making careful notes. Eighteen months later, David attended the practice for a check-up. The dentist was unable to detect any changes in the quality of the bone surrounding the apex of UL1. It was no better but had not got any worse.

David plays rugby at quite a high level, so at each visit the dentist adjured him to wear the mouth guard he had made for him. David admits that he does not always do so as, he says, he cannot breathe well with it in, and the 'lads' cannot understand what he shouts to them when there is a lineout. The dentist feels obliged to warn him that he has very expensive dentistry in his mouth and that a blow to a post crown would undoubtedly cause loss of the tooth.

David is not keen to wear the mouth guard. The dentist has recommended that he wears it because of the negative consequences that could accrue should he not follow advice. The use of negative consequences is one method of attempting to gain attention and acceptance by the patient so that he/she will adhere to recommendations. What does the literature say about successfully motivating patients using this approach of appeal to fear? There is extensive research, dating back to the 1950s, on the effect on patients of adopting frightening or shocking messages. It is difficult to say what is the best way of persuading the patient to embark on a programme that requires his/her cooperation and adherence to recommendations. A key factor for the dentist to ascertain is the extent to which the patient believes that they can follow through with the dentist's recommendations. This is known as perceived efficacy. If, for example, the patient has very little capacity to follow the recommendations that you wish the patient to adhere to, then a frightening message may only succeed in encouraging the patient to develop a 'tough shell' and hence ignore your advice. For patients who are confident in their ability to act, because they have the means to adopt the measure, either financially or because they have sufficient time, then there is good evidence that fear-appeal can be very effective in raising the perceived threat and therefore promoting behavioural change. The dentist therefore needs to be sensitive to the beliefs that patients hold about how confident they are about following advice. Practical suggestions which are tailored to the individual patient and which increase a patient's confidence in adhering to the advice often help to produce good outcomes. However, this can be coupled with supplying a message of negative consequences if the patient continues to vacillate, remains at 'status quo', or continues not to follow the professional advice.

A further approach which has been found to encourage behavioural adherence is to assess the patient's willingness to act differently. In other words the dentist needs to assess whether the patient feels ready to change. Once this has been established, then the dentist can determine how to proceed. Should the patient feel that they are simply too busy at present, or that they don't feel the recommended action fits into their lifestyle, the dentist might make a note in the patient's record to ask again about their 'readiness to change'. The dentist might try to leave the patient with a message tailored to the patient's own beliefs about their condition and could also describe the positive consequences of changing their behaviour. This consistent and longer-term approach can be effective but requires careful note taking and the use of negotiating skills with the patient. The term 'motivational interviewing' is applied to this structured, cumulative, and patient-centred approach and is widely used in tobacco smoking cessation programmes. It is interesting that David did sometimes wear the mouth guard at the rugby match, so maybe the message imparted to David by the dentist had some influence after all.

A week and a half later, David attends the surgery again. He is off-colour and in incredible pain from UL1. He said that he wore his mouth guard at his last rugby match but had been punched in the face at least twice during the game. David could not bear UL1 to be touched and he said that he has been unable to either eat or sleep since Sunday night (3 days ago).

Aggressively, David demands that the dentist get him out of pain. The dentist explained that it would be difficult to achieve adequate anaesthesia for extracting the tooth or in order to undertake any other type of treatment.

David begs again for the dentist to do something and yet he cannot bear have the tooth or surrounding mucosa touched. A radiograph (taken with difficulty) showed pretty much the same appearance as the previous two, which were taken at David's check-ups. The dentist feels under terrible pressure to take the tooth out, as David is so upset, and is desperate for the source of the pain to be removed.

You have a duty of care to this patient and therefore must undertake a full history and examination, including radiographs, to exclude bone and tooth/root fractures.

You establish that the pain was definitely emanating from the periapical area of UL1, but there was no radiographic evidence of either a bone or root fracture. Your treatment options are, therefore:

1. You could refer David to the oral surgery department of the nearest district general hospital, with a request that they deal with David's pain.
2. You could attempt to obtain anaesthesia via an intra-orbital block and supplementary infiltration anaesthesia and remove the tooth.
3. As for option 2 but then remove the crown and the post and try to achieve drainage through the root in order to relieve David's pain.
4. You could give David antibiotics and analgesics and ask him to come back in 3 days' time when you will attempt to drain the UL1 as per option 3 but without local anaesthetic.

The first option is really only the treatment of choice if none of the other treatment modalities will suffice to make the patient's pain bearable. It is also perhaps worth keeping in mind that David, while in severe pain, is not perhaps able to clearly think through the longer-term consequences of any of the treatment options. However, he is a patient who has previously sued a dentist because a root treatment was not well performed.

The question that arises here is one of diminished autonomy, possibly caused by pain of such an intensity that David is incompetent in respect of decision-making about treatment for UL1. It is not for the dentist to try to consider what David would have chosen were he not in pain. Although this type of pain can be very severe and debilitating it would not be sufficient to incapacitate David from any proper decision-making if extraction was performed.

Removal of the tooth would give immediate relief from pain. All of the other options to relieve the pain therefore need careful explanation. Once the tooth was removed replacement would not be too difficult, either by fixed bridgework or possibly an implant. All these options and the benefits of trying to keep the tooth would need discussion. Following such a full discussion David would be able to arrive, despite the pain, at a fully 'informed choice', even if that choice was extraction.

A general anaesthetic is anyway always a last resort as it carries with it a quantifiable risk of death. Thus, if the tooth is to be extracted, it would usually be taken out under simple infiltration local anaesthesia. However, David appeared to have a spreading infection and inflammation and it is therefore not advisable to inject into the inflamed/infected area. Block anaesthesia can overcome such difficulties, but it should be recognized that with exquisitely tender-to-touch teeth such as David's it is sometimes very difficult to obtain sufficient anaesthesia for extraction with local anaesthetic. The arguments against extraction per se apply as much to extractions under local anaesthesia as to extractions under general anaesthesia, i.e. patients in very severe pain may not be competent to give informed consent.

The third option is a good option if David feels he is willing to try to save the root of the tooth and if sufficient anaesthesia can be achieved. If this is possible, the tooth should be left on open drainage and antibiotics should be prescribed.

The fourth option is a sort of 'holding' option and does not address the patient's expressed demands, nor does it provide immediate relief for the intense pain the patient is suffering.

After much discussion about the options, David agrees that, although he desperately wishes to be out of pain and wants the tooth removed, he would have the crown removed and keep the tooth root.

Up to 10% of treatments may have to be abandoned owing to failure of local anaesthesia. Failure may be most apparent in the management of endodontically involved teeth. Difficulties in obtaining anaesthesia may be overcome by:

- giving more solution (up to 2 ml per 10 kg of body weight),
- giving a different solution, such as articaine,
- using a different technique, e.g. intraligamentary injections or nerve blocks (as opposed to infiltration anaesthesia).

Using an appropriate anaesthetic technique the crown was removed by cutting it off with a burr. The post was then removed using an ultrasonic tip and drainage through the tooth achieved, giving David substantial relief from his pain. Once the acute infection subsided, a well-condensed root filling was placed in the apical third of the root and a post core and crown provided. The shade was carefully chosen in consultation with David and he appeared to be very happy with the result. However, 12 months later, David presented again with pain from the same tooth.

On radiographing the tooth, although the root filling looked extremely good, a well-defined radiolucency, approximately 0.75 cm in diameter, with a rim of well condensed bone, was visible. This was diagnosed as a cyst. The only sensible option at this stage was to perform periradicular surgery.

Indications for apicectomy

- The presence of periradicular disease in a root-filled tooth where conventional root canal treatment cannot be undertaken or has failed, or where conventional re-treatment may be detrimental to retention of the tooth.
- Presence of periradicular disease in a tooth where iatrogenic or developmental anomalies prevent conventional root canal treatment.
- Where a biopsy of periradicular tissue is required.
- Where visualization of the periradicular tissues and tooth root is required when perforation, root crack, or fracture is suspected.
- Where procedures are required that require either tooth sectioning or root amputation.
- Where it may not be expedient to undertake prolonged non-surgical root canal treatment because of patient considerations.

In this case, the only sensible option for preserving the tooth is an apicectomy. It is of course not the only option. The tooth could be extracted, but it would seem that David is now keen to save the tooth. Without discussion of all the options David will not have made an informed choice about the treatment he undergoes in respect of the cyst. David most certainly needs to be made aware of the prospects for a successful outcome, and that there can be no guarantees of success in any clinical treatment. Even if the treatment fails, provided that the apicectomy is performed to acceptable clinical standards, the dentist would be supported by the law.

David asked whether the periradicular surgery procedure would give him a really good chance of keeping his tooth and the dentist said that it would.

The success rates of periradicular surgery is between 30 and 80%. However, if further surgery is required (i.e. the treatment does not work), the chance of a second operation being successful is around 35%.

The periradicular surgery was duly performed and the cyst curetted out. On inspection, during the periradicular surgery, the seal at the root face appeared to be sound so no retrograde root filling was placed.

Procedure for apicectomy

- Where possible, use a local anaesthetic that includes a haemostatic agent such as epinephrine.
- The use of an operating microscope has been shown to be of benefit.
- Lift a full-thickness flap extended to the gingival sulcus or with a scalloped submarginal incision.

- If bone removal is necessary, this should be carried out with a burr cooled with sterile water or saline.
- Curette out any inflammatory tissue.
- Root end resection should remove at least 3 mm of the root and should be as close to 90° to the long axis of the tooth as possible.
- Root end preparation should be carried out using an ultrasonic tip or burr in a miniature head handpiece. The tip or burr should be cooled. The preparation should be 3 mm deep.
- Mineral trioxide aggregate (MTA), super EBA, glass ionomer, composite resin, and reinforced zinc oxide eugenol are the most suitable root end filling materials.
- Close with sutures.
- Remove sutures after 48–96 h.

The healing after the procedure was uneventful. However, 3 weeks and two courses of antibiotics later, David was still experiencing symptoms from the tooth.

The treatment options at this stage were:

1. Repeat the surgery on the tooth.
2. Extract the tooth and replace with: an implant; a conventional bridge; a resin retained bridge; a cobalt-chrome denture; or nothing.

Option 1 is a possibility but the chances of success diminish each time a tooth is apicectomized. Given that David had hoped for a positive outcome from the first procedure and had then experienced a negative one, it is unlikely that he would, if given this information, wish to proceed. Indeed, when the odds of success are explained to David, he becomes angry and seeks a second opinion, saying he will sue if he has been 'messed up'.

To manage angry patients:

- First, ensure that you are in a private room and only you, the patient, and your ancillary staff, if present, can hear your conversation. If you are in the surgery then ensure that privacy is maintained by closing the door.
- Second, do not react with anger yourself but stay calm.
- Third, acknowledge as best you can, what the patient is trying to convey so that the patient is convinced that you see their problem from their point of view (example: Yes, I can see that you are in great discomfort with this tooth, this is very upsetting, and also that you are very keen to try and resolve your pain. Here are the options that we can offer...).
- Fourth, reward the patient by thanking them for their honesty or the fact that he/she is a respected client of the practice and you will do everything you can to try and resolve their problem.

It should be a policy of the practice that harassment and discrimination within the practice should not be tolerated. If patients do complain about the way they have been treated then this needs to be investigated seriously. However, if the patient becomes abusive or offensive and a member of staff determines the behaviour to be 'inappropriate' then the patient needs to be told, as an informal warning, that their behaviour is unacceptable. A formal warning needs to be made should the behaviour continue. Depending on the policy of the practice there may be case to de-register the patient. It is hoped that the adoption of the methods outlined above would prevent the need for such warnings to be made. However, the NHS has a zero-tolerance policy on harassment and details are available from their website. It is especially pertinent with minority ethnic group staff working in the NHS. Respondents to an NHS survey reported that harassment by patients is most commonly in the form of verbal abuse. The Department of Health has issued guidance for Trusts on circumstances where patients consistently refuse treatment from staff of different ethnic origin.

However, having visited two further dentists, who offered him similar treatment, David returns to your surgery, apologizing for his behaviour and anger, and asks whether you would remove the tooth and place an implant.

It would seem that David has revealed why he sought treatment from you for a replacement crown all that time ago. His last dentist probably refused to treat him again, and ended up being sued.

David is, of course, entitled to seek such a second opinion. Further, the dentist ought to have suggested that David seek a second opinion and even made a referral. David has received two opinions that seem to support the first dentist's view. Rather unusually he has returned to the dentist asking her/him for further treatment. He is obviously satisfied that the dentist is competent.

Does the dentist have to take him back? If he is a registered NHS patient and no request was made to de-register him when he threatened legal action then it may take up to 3 months to de-register him, with a requirement to provide emergency treatment in the interim. If he is a private patient then the choice is yours.

The dentist agrees to undertake the treatment and, after a long discussion with David about the pros and cons of such treatment, places a single tooth implant.

For several years after the fitting of the single tooth implant, David attends regularly for check-ups and treatment when required. He has one or two pieces of conventional restorative work done but nothing major. David then stops attending and nothing is heard of him for 4 years.

The dentist then received a letter from a casualty department:

Dear

Mr David Lester has been attending this casualty department for treatment of a broken left mandible which he sustained in a fight in Anytown Rugby Club. The police were involved and legal action may result from their enquiries.

In the meantime, whilst David was under our treatment for the fracture, it was noted that he required some routine dental treatment. He gave your name as his dentist and we are therefore writing so that you are aware of the fracture which was treated using two finger plates, and of the circumstances in which the injuries were sustained.

Yours sincerely

Several days later, David rings for a dental appointment. When he attends, he complains of pain in the joint of his jaw on the right-hand side. He also needs two restorations. These are carried out but David continues to complain about the pain in his 'jaw joint'. His occlusion seems no different from previously and no signs of temporomandibular joint (TMJ) disease (click, muscle tenderness, deviation) can be detected.

David says that the pain is so bad that he cannot work. He asks the dentist if he will come to court and say that the pain was due to the injuries he sustained in the fight.

It seems that, following the assault, David has some TMJ problems. However, the dentist cannot detect any of the usual clinical signs or any abnormalities. In such circumstances, the dentist should not agree to say that the pain the patient is suffering was caused by the injuries sustained in the fight. It is the dentist's professional opinion that there are no TMJ problems, and if he attends Court, this is what he must say. However, it is unlikely in either criminal proceedings or civil proceedings that the dentist would be called to give evidence. In criminal proceedings the fact of the fracture as ascertained by the hospital records would be sufficient for the Crown Prosecution to determine the level of charges to be brought against David's assailant. In civil proceedings the dentist could be called to act as a witness of fact as to injuries received and treatment required in consequence. It seems that there were no dental injuries *per se*, and in those circumstances the hospital records ought to suffice. However, David's assertion of continuing pain in his TMJ is perhaps a matter which requires expert opinion, particularly as the dentist is unable to diagnose any problem. Such expert opinion would not normally be taken from the treating dentist, and David, as he well knows, requires an expert witness who can give the court opinion in addition to fact. In any event, most certainly the dentist would be advised to make an appropriate referral to determine whether there are or are not any TMJ problems.

BIBLIOGRAPHY

British Dental Association. *Supporting Colleagues: Dealing with Harassment of the Dental Team by Patients*. BDA advice sheet D16. British Dental Association: London, 2003.

Brunton PA. *Decision-Making in Operative Dentistry*. Quintessence: London, 2002.

Kay EJ, Blinkhorn AS. Some factors related to dentists' decisions to extract teeth. *Community Dental Health* 1987; **4**: 3–8.

Kay EJ, Nuttall NM. *Clinical Decision Making. An Art or a Science*. BDJ Books: London, 1995.

Kent G. Memory of dental pain. *Pain* 1985; **21**: 187–194.

Meechan JG. *Practical Dental Local Anaesthesia*. Quintessence: London, 2002.

NHSE. *Campaign to Stop Violence Against Staff Working in the NHS: NHS Zero Tolerance Zone*, HSC 1999/226. Leeds: NHSE, 1999. www.nhs.uk/zerotolerance/intro.htm

Petersen PE, Holst D. Utilization of dental health services. In: Cohen LK, Gift HC (eds) *Disease Prevention and Oral Health Promotion*, pp 341–386. Munksgaard: Copenhagen, 1995.

Ray HA, Trope M. Periapical status of endodontically treated teeth in relation to the technical quality of the root filling and the coronal restoration. *International Endodontics Journal* 1995; **28**: 12–18.

Shearer A, Mellor A. *Treatment Planning in Primary Dental Care*. Oxford University Press: Oxford, 2003.

Stephenson MT, Witte K. Fear, threat, and perception of efficacy from frightening skin cancer messages. *Public Health Review* 1998; **26**(2):147–174.

The Royal College of Surgeons of England. *Guidelines for Surgical Endodontics*. www.rcseng.ac.uk/dental/fds/pdf/surg_end_guideline.pdf

4 Kylie: a nervous mum

Kylie is a feisty 20-year-old woman who is pregnant. She attends a dental surgery after recently moving into the area. She has a heavily restored dentition with all her posterior teeth containing amalgams. UR1, UL2 are crowned and UL1 has large and badly discoloured composite restorations. The lower anterior teeth have new cavities, which fortunately are not yet extensive. Her oral hygiene is good, but on questioning her diet is revealed to be highly cariogenic. She drinks six to eight cups of sweetened tea during the day (she takes three teaspoonfuls of sugar in each) and three to four carbonated soft drinks in the evening. The dentist asks about her smoking habits and she says she smokes approximately five cigarettes per day but does not drink alcohol.

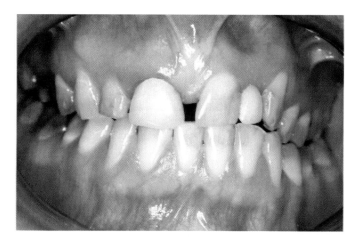

Heavily restored anterior teeth

Is it important to ask people about their smoking habits?
Should the dentist give smoking advice?

Kylie lives alone, on state benefit, in a council-owned property. She says that she occasionally sings in clubs and bars to supplement her income. She seems to swing between being delighted and excited by her pregnancy and being extremely angry about it. There is no indication that she is in a long-term relationship with her baby's father. She complains rather a lot about the poor standard of living which the state provides for her and is looking forward to the extra income the baby will bring to her household.

How do Kylie's social circumstances and background influence her response to dentists?

What is 'locus of control' and 'locus of responsibility' and how do they affect Kylie?

Kylie complains of a bit of toothache at the back of her mouth. She says it only hurts when she bites hard on the left-hand side of her mouth. When the dentist examines Kylie's mouth, he sees that the LL6 has an amalgam in it, with extensive recurrent caries.

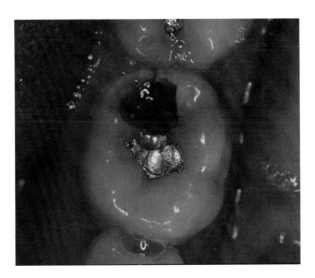

Recurrent caries in LL6

Despite this history of mild toothache, Kylie's chief concern is that she wants a new appearance for her front teeth. As she puts it, she needs to look 'different'. The dentist assumes this desire is related to her singing career. She demands (rather than asks) that the dentist crown her teeth.

How can the dentist successfully relate to the patient when an inappropriate treatment option is sought by the patient?

Kylie then says that she does not want a white but a gold crown on UR2. She insists that she is eligible for such treatment on the National Health Service, but says she will, if she has to, pay to have a gold, rather than tooth-coloured crown.

Can the dentist provide this crown on the NHS?

Is it ethical to provide this treatment?

Radiographs of Kylie's teeth are taken. Bitewings, and periapicals UR2, UR1, UL1, UL2, and LL6 show a periapical radiolucency on the mesial root of LL6.

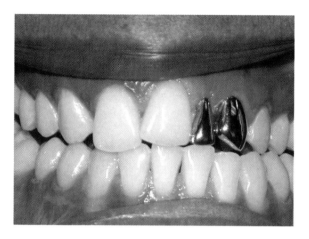

Metal anterior crowns

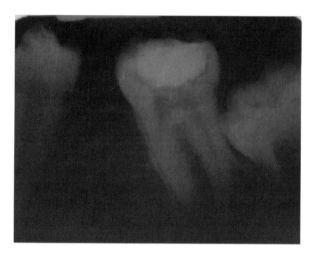

Periradicular periodontitis in a LL6

Is it permissible to take these radiographs when the patient is pregnant?
How can a tooth exhibit signs of both vitality and non-vitality?
Diagnosis

High caries rate with:

1. Mesial and distal caries LR2, LR1, LL1, LL2.
2. Periradicular periodontitis mesial root LL6.
3. Poor appearance UR1, UL1, UL2.

The most pressing concern from the dentist's point of view is to relieve Kylie's pain, although this is not necessarily Kylie's priority. The dentist considers removing the amalgam and placing a sedative dressing. But instead, he opts to extract the tooth at a future visit. Kylie agrees to this course of action.

Is this treatment appropriate, ethically, legally, and clinically?

The dentist explains that Kylie will then need to return for restoration of the lower anterior teeth after the LL6 has been extracted and after that, perhaps, for a crown on UL1 to improve appearance. The dentist does not mention the gold crown for UR2. He does, however, try to explain the process for making and fitting crowns, but Kylie waves his explanations aside, saying she 'knows how it's done, she's had them before'.

Should treatment proceed?

Second visit: Kylie attends for her extraction. She says the tooth has been worse since the last visit and has woken her up in the night on three occasions.

Why do patients often complain that their toothache is worse at night?

Kylie says she has had to take strong painkillers in order to cope with the pain of the toothache.

Kylie is not anxious or nervous about either injection or extractions so the dentist proceeds in the normal way. Two minutes after the administration of the inferior alveolar block, Kylie reports that both her lip and tongue are numb on the left-hand side. The block is supplemented with a long buccal nerve injection. Anaesthesia is checked by probing round the tooth, then the socket expanded using an elevator. Kylie appears to be quite happy and comfortable during these processes.

Finally the forceps are placed on the tooth and the dentist proceeds to extract the tooth.

What is known about the relationship of anxiety and pain?
What is the technique for extracting lower molar teeth?

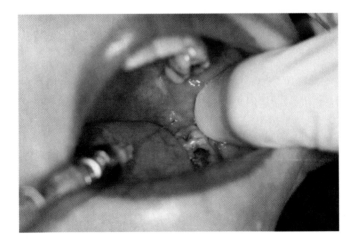

Inferior dental block injection

Suddenly Kylie shrieks for the dentist to stop. She is crying and says that it hurts 'like hell', as she puts it. The dentist explains patiently that if her tongue, lip, and gums are numb she cannot possibly feel pain from the extraction.

Is pain a subjective or objective experience?

The dentist tells her that if she did not feel the elevator then the tooth is anaesthetized and that all she is feeling is pressure. After a while, Kylie settles down and appears to have accepted the dentist's interpretation of the situation.

Why can the tooth extraction precipitate such a strong reaction in a patient?

Once again, the forceps are placed on the tooth and the extraction attempted. Once more, just as the tooth moves significantly in the socket, Kylie yells. This time, she pushes the dentist away and leaps to her feet. She shouts that the dentist is a dangerous and incompetent man, and runs out of the door.

Has the dentist acted appropriately? If not, what has he done wrong?
Could/should the dentist give more local anaesthetic, and how could it be given?
What effect is this event likely to have on Kylie's ability to accept dentistry?

Five weeks later, Kylie presents at a second dentist. She presents looking completely terrified and asking/begging to see a female dentist. She says that her boyfriend will pay privately for any treatment she has.

Can the dentist agree to a third party paying for an individual's treatment?

Kylie has come to the surgery because UR1 has been knocked out, apparently during the course of a domestic dispute. Kylie does not say who was responsible for the injuries to her teeth but the new dentist assumes that it must have been the father of Kylie's unborn child.

What should the dentist do about this suspected assault?
How common is domestic violence and what is its effect?

Kylie does not have the avulsed tooth and the incident apparently happened 2 days ago.

Under what circumstances can teeth be replanted?

The female dentist agrees to construct an acrylic denture for Kylie but advises her that, so long as her oral hygiene remains good, other more permanent solutions might be possible. Kylie states that she will not have any treatment other than the denture, as she 'does not trust' dentists.

How can trust be restored in patients who have had a traumatic dental experience?

However, when the denture is delivered, Kylie is so relieved and pleased with her improved appearance that she becomes a little more relaxed. The dentist

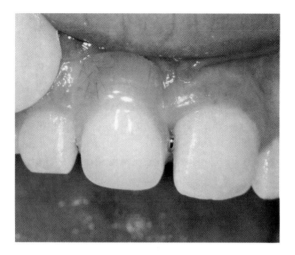

Denture replacing an UR1

takes time to explain that the fit of the denture will change as the gums remodel, and that she will need a new denture, or an alternative, within the near future.

Why will Kylie need a new denture so soon?

Kylie promises to attend every 6 months after the birth of her child, which is now due in 2 months' time.

At each of Kylie's subsequent visits, Kylie's confidence in the dentist grows but she claims she cannot and will not have any treatment which involves injections or potential pain 'unless she is knocked out'.

How does this relate to Kylie's previous experience?

After 2 years the nurse finally manages to persuade Kylie to have her teeth radiographed and a large periapical radiolucency is visible, associated with UL1. The dentist explains that root treatment is required in order to make sure that symptoms do not arise. Kylie asks: '... if there's a problem, why doesn't it hurt'? When the dentist argues that it *may* hurt in the future, Kylie asks what percentage of teeth like her UL1 start to hurt. In the end Kylie says that she will attend to have the tooth treated if it begins to hurt.

How should Kylie's questions be answered?
Should all patients participate in decision-making?

A further 2 years later Kylie attends again, with her 4-year-old child. She has been experiencing problems with the UL1, but is still extremely fearful of treatment. She explains that this is so because of the dentist who hurt her, nearly 5 years ago. She explains how she had to go to hospital to have the tooth which he had loosened taken out under general anaesthetic, but that the experience with the dentist, who would not take any notice of her screams, was the worst thing that ever happened to her, and that she now cannot ever trust anyone to put any sort of instrument in her mouth.

Is Kylie 'phobic' of dentistry?

The dentist then offers treatment to Kylie under inhalation sedation, explains that no injections will be needed, and talks to Kylie about stop signals.

Is inhalation sedation an appropriate treatment modality?
What is the procedure and why are stop signals necessary?

After a number of acclimatization visits, at which Kylie is slowly introduced to treatment, Kylie copes well with the root canal treatment of UL1. Having gained some confidence she then requests that you place a gold crown on this tooth. She also says that the denture carrying UR1 is causing her great embarrassment when she sings, as it drops down sometimes.

What are the areas of oral functioning that patients may rate as vital to their overall quality of life?

Treatment options

Kylie has a reasonably intact but heavily restored dentition and has UR1 missing. UL1 is root filled and heavily restored, UL2 is crowned, UR2 is sound.

The options to replace UR1 that should be discussed with Kylie are:

- Another denture—in either acrylic or cobalt chrome: This is the most retrievable situation as no or minimal tooth preparation would be required. Dentures can also replace bone and soft tissue as well as teeth, and if there had been significant resorption then this may be a good option. However, the risks of partial dentures include increased plaque and caries levels and increased numbers of root surface restorations. Kylie has managed to wear the partial denture, which was fitted immediately following the loss of the tooth, and there will have been bone resorption since that time resulting in loss of stability and retention of the denture. If she were provided with a better-fitting and more retentive denture then she may cope quite well.
- Resin-retained bridge: If the UL1 were sound and the occlusion favourable this would be a strong contender for restoring the UR1 space. However, the large restorations in the UL1 would be difficult to replace or repair if they failed when a resin-retained bridge was in place.
- Conventional bridge: When there are heavily restored teeth adjacent to the missing tooth/teeth, then a conventional bridge becomes a likely option. In Kylie's case it may be possible to cantilever the UR1 pontic from a retainer on the UL1.
- Implant: An implant would be possible in this situation although if Kylie still smokes this may be considered a contraindication to implant provision. Other concerns are the long-term prognosis for Kylie's remaining upper anterior teeth, as the UL1 and UL2 are heavily restored and UL1 is root filled.

Kylie opts for an acrylic denture as she feels this will suit her best and she can always go for another of the options at a later date. The dentist suggests to Kylie that she bring her daughter along with her when she comes for her appointments.

KYLIE: A NERVOUS MUM

Kylie is a feisty 20-year-old woman who is pregnant. She attends a dental surgery after recently moving into the area. She has a heavily restored dentition with all her posterior teeth containing amalgams. UR1, UL2 are crowned and UL1 has large and badly discoloured composite restorations. The lower anterior teeth have new cavities, which fortunately are not yet extensive. Her oral hygiene is good, but on questioning her diet is revealed to be highly cariogenic. She drinks six to eight cups of sweetened tea during the day (she takes three teaspoonfuls of sugar in each) and three to four carbonated soft drinks in the evening. The dentist asks about her smoking habits and she says she smokes approximately five cigarettes per day but does not drink alcohol.

In the UK about 28% of the adult population smoke. Increasingly, smokers belong to the lower socioeconomic sectors of society. Smoking tobacco not only carries general health risks, such as increased risk of heart disease, lung cancer, and respiratory illnesses, but it is also related to periodontal disease, oral cancer, and the success of implants.

Asking a patient whether or not they smoke, and if so, how many cigarettes they smoke, provides relevant information for the dental practitioner but also opens the door towards offering advice on quitting the habit. If Kylie had smoked more than 20 cigarettes in a day, and if she lit her first one within 30 minutes of waking in the morning, she would be classified as heavily dependent and such people will have great difficulty in quitting. However, Kylie only smokes (or says she only smokes) five cigarettes each day, and these are always smoked in the evening, so stopping the habit should be relatively easy for her.

All patients who smoke should be advised of the health and oral health risks related to their habit. Not only are there strong detrimental effects on general health, such as increased risk of lung cancer, and stroke, but also oral health problems are exacerbated including periodontal disease, leucoplakia, and oral cancer. Stained teeth and halitosis are often powerful motivators for stopping for younger people. These things are often more personally relevant to them than, say, the threat of compromised lung function later in their life.

Smokers who seek dental care should, as a matter of routine, be asked about their smoking habits. The dentist has a duty to provide patients with information about the options available to them. Dentists can be of assistance to their patients by recognizing the oral signs of tobacco use and draw the patient's attention to them. The dentist can ask at this point about willingness to quit. If they express a wish to quit, the dentist should be able to offer appropriate help and support by referring to local smoking cessation services. Nagging or insisting that people quit when they have no desire to simply wastes time and also increases resistance to further invitations to quit at a later date. The provision of advice from the dentist and other members of the dental team can, on repeated visits over time, encourage the patient to consider moving from a stage of not wishing to quit (pre-contemplation), to possible intention to quit (contemplation), to actual setting of a quit date (action) and eventually quitting (maintenance). This model is now familiar to many in the smoking cessation field and is known as the 'trans-theoretical model of behaviour change'. It is an important aid for health-care personnel as it helps to explain that not all people are ready to change and it may require a few attempts by the dental team to encourage some movement towards the goal of quitting. However, it is vital that the team do not pressurize the individual but gently encourage and match the reason that the patient volunteers to contemplate or take action with some well chosen words, advice, and support. Dentists can prescribe nicotine replacement therapy and an NHS Smoker's Helpline is available (0800 169 0 169) to offer advice in English and Welsh. Dentists are recommended to ring Quitline to gain information on support services for patients who speak other languages (0800 00 2200). The four As model is a helpful framework in this field of persuading patients to stop smoking. It includes:

• Asking about smoking and their desire to stop.
• Advice about the benefits of quitting.
• Assisting the patient to stop through access to appropriate support.
• Arranging follow-up support.

Even brief advice (2 minutes) given to patients about stopping smoking will help an additional 2% of smokers per year to successfully stop smoking. This figure can be raised to 6% if more intensive support, plus nicotine replacement therapy, is given.

Therefore, if all dentists offered advice on stopping smoking, around an extra 100 000 smokers might quit. Barriers to introducing smoking cessation advice routinely include: lack of confidence in the dental personnel's ability to encourage behaviour change, smoking habits of health-care staff themselves, and lack of time. As has been mentioned previously, even a small intervention lasting about 2 minutes can produce measurable long-term effects, and dental teams can develop close ties with local smoking cessation services to supply more intensive and sophisticated interventions.

Kylie lives alone, on state benefit, in a council-owned property. She says that she occasionally sings in clubs and bars to supplement her income. She seems to swing between being delighted and excited by her pregnancy and being extremely angry about it. There is no indication that she is in a long-term relationship with her baby's father. She complains rather a lot about the poor standard of living which the state provides for her and is looking forward to the extra income the baby will bring to her household.

Kylie as head of household in her council accommodation would probably be classified (being part-time performing artist) as social class III (NM) in the Registrar General's classification of occupational types. She would be considered as skilled non-manual. The classification has five social classes (from I 'Professional' to V 'Unskilled') and this scale is used in national dental surveys. The category III is split into NM, skilled non-manual, and M, skilled manual. The category assigned to an individual is the occupational status of the head of household. The scale can be helpful to give an approximate estimate of the likely differences in oral health, behaviour, and attitudes that might be expected with patients from the different categories. A note of caution should be made not to take this predicted profile for each social class too literally, as within each social class there is wide individual variation. However, attendance rates tend to be lower for social classes III, IV, and V. Hence Kylie may not be as regular an attender as those from social classes I and II. This generalization may not be borne out by an examination of Kylie's mouth, which indicates substantial dental treatment in the past and good oral hygiene. The dentist would need to be careful not to pre-judge the patient with the background knowledge that was available, (expectant single mother living in a council flat). It is known from a national survey that regardless of social class, women tend to be less satisfied with their dental treatment than men (19% compared with 15%), hence social class, although helpful from a public viewpoint to study inequalities, is less useful when treating individuals where a more comprehensive approach should be made to assessing suitability for prevention and treatment programmes.

'Locus of control' is the degree to which each of us believes we control what happens to us. Those with high *internal* locus of control believe that if they behave in certain ways, certain 'rewards' or good outcomes will happen. For example, you probably believe that if you work hard at your exams, you are more likely to be successful in them.

However, some people with *external* locus of control believe that luck, or chance, is the most powerful influence over what happens to them, whilst others again will believe that what ultimately happens is in the hands of a 'powerful other'. This might be their god, or the government, or perhaps a parent or spouse.

People who are of low socioeconomic status, and women, often have external rather than internal loci of control. This is unsurprising, because if a male partner, or local government, or pure economics tend to influence how your life is, rather than your own personal choices influencing it, then you are highly likely to have an external locus of control.

Of course people will have a different (health) locus of control (HLOC) in different situations, and at different time points, but HLOC is a way of describing people's beliefs about control, and power. It refers to one's beliefs about the degree of control one has over external events and over the behaviour of others. It is important to recognize that the HLOC concept does *not* refer to a person's beliefs about their ability to manage their *own* behaviour.

So, HLOC is what a person believes about who or what *can* influence health. A further concept describes people's beliefs about who or what *should* be doing something about their health. This second concept is known as Health Locus of Responsibility (HLOR).

'Locus of responsibility' refers to the degree to which 'blame' for one's circumstances, or in the case of HLOR, one's health, is placed on the individual or on the 'system'.

Kylie shows by her complaints that she feels the 'system' is responsible for her standard of living, and, to some extent, for her baby. She therefore clearly has an external locus of responsibility. However, her oral hygiene is good. If she brushes for the sake of her oral health, her cleanliness would suggest that she has an internal HLOC. This is important. If a person believes that some one, or something, else controls how their health turns out, they are unlikely to take actions to benefit their health. Therefore, health education is likely to be more successful with people with an internal health locus of control. People with an external health locus of control believe that their health is controlled by, perhaps, the health system, or their dentist, or even the environment or luck. They are therefore less likely to take action on behalf of their health. Ultimately, they believe that they do not control it, and therefore it is pointless to try to influence one's health by behaving in certain ways. These beliefs can be highly stable and require time and encouragement to change. The processes involved are not always clear-cut and substantial variation is found across individuals. Dentists should have some understanding of the possible belief structures that people hold, in order that the advice offered to patients is not so systematic that it ignores the patient's views. A consequence of an overly standardized manner from the dentist is that it sends a message that the dentist is insensitive and bases his/her contact with patients in a mechanistic approach, which can cause alienatation.

Kylie complains of a bit of toothache at the back of her mouth. She says it only hurts when she bites hard on the left-hand side of her mouth. When the dentist examines Kylie's mouth, he sees that the LL6 has a very large amalgam in it, with extensive recurrent caries.

Despite this history of mild toothache, Kylie's chief concern is that she wants a new appearance for her front teeth. As she puts it, she needs to look 'different'. The dentist assumes this desire is related to her singing career. She demands (rather than asks) that the dentist crown her teeth.

It is one of the challenges to the dentist to engage their patients and help deliver to them high-quality dental care. There are at least three types of clinician–patient relationship: paternalistic, mutualistic, and consumerist. The latter could be stated as the modern approach to service delivery in health services. Patients request different opinions about their treatment planning and consider their requirements according to what can be met from within a market place with ample levels of detailed information. Decisions can then be made to select the service they wish to conduct their treatment. However, patients will vary in their wish to make decisions about treatment. In a paternalistic relationship the patient is advised that the dentist will give information about various treatments available and suggest a suitable plan for the patient. Alternatively, the dentist can state that the patient can have a greater say in the treatment so that the dentist enters into a partnership with the patient in their joint discussion of the treatment options. This may be an ideal, as in reality the dentist will have considerably advanced knowledge compared to the patient. However, the patient may feel that they are the 'expert' about their own body and may insist that they have the final say, even if this is contrary to the dentist's opinion. The dentist should determine early on in the relationship with the patient how the patient would prefer to receive their dental care.

Kylie's views are clearly at odds with the dentist and emotions for both parties appear to be rapidly raised. Recent research from Sweden with patients receiving prosthetic dental treatments has clearly shown from detailed video records and transcripts of the communication processes between patients and dentists, that a significant component of the interactions between dentists and their patients consists of emotional material such as patients conveying concern, expressing direct disapproval, and seeking reassurance. Hence, although the process of fitting implants and dentures has a very technical aspect, it is clear that there are emotional exchanges which require the dentist to encourage expression by the patient in order to reduce any build-up of resentment or feeling of distress and discomfort.

Kylie then says that she does not want a white but a gold crown on UR2. She insists that she is eligible for such treatment on the National Health Service, but says she will, if she has to, pay to have a gold, rather than tooth-coloured crown.

The request for and provision of gold crowns on anterior teeth is not unusual in some cultures and communities. If there is a clinical requirement for a crown then whether the crown provided is a gold crown, or any other colour, there is no reason not to accede to a patient's request for such a crown. It goes without saying that such treatment should only be provided after discussing fully with the patient all the other available treatment options, risks and benefits, etc. In the usual way it would be important to tell the patient that the average life expectancy of a crown would be about 12–15 years. However, because it is possible that the patient may request a replacement sooner (they may tire of their 'different' appearance as they get older), it is probably important to also tell the patient that each cycle of replacement carries a risk of further tooth destruction and tooth tissue loss and a risk of some detriment to the tooth. The NHS would not provide for a gold crown on an anterior tooth. However, the dentist could check this, and could reassure Kylie that he was doing his best by making an application and seeking approval in the normal way.

To illustrate the arguments that arise in the provision of treatment for which there is no clinical need, but which is requested to effect a change in appearance, it is better to assume that the tooth is currently of satisfactory appearance. Such treatment could not be provided by the NHS. It would have to be provided privately.

The ethical arguments against providing a crown simply to change someone's appearance are that there would be unnecessary and irreversible destruction of sound tooth tissue. The crown preparation would carry the risk of loss of vitality and the need for root canal treatment and therefore a potential risk of periapical infection, fracture of the tooth, and ultimately a possible risk of tooth loss. These risks are always associated with crown preparation. It could be argued that the probability of such risks materializing would be less in a sound healthy tooth as there have been no previous 'assaults on the pulp'. The risks would, however, be exactly the same as those faced when preparing a tooth for a crown because it is discoloured, if there were no pathological basis for such discoloration.

Given such a clinical scenario it would appear that most dentists would have no concerns in providing a tooth-coloured crown (assuming a veneer to be contraindicated) to improve aesthetics. This would restore the appearance of the patient's teeth to that perceived as normal and acceptable by society in general and by the dentist. Most dentists would probably agree that provided the patient was 'fully informed' such treatment would be considered ethical.

However, if the patient wishes to alter the appearance of a front tooth, which was already perceived as normal by the dentist and society, this would create some ethical dissonance. Most dentists would probably consider it unethical to accede to such a request.

This a matter of balance between some of the principles of health-care ethics, namely:

• autonomy
• non-maleficence—do no harm
• beneficence—do good.

The vast majority of health-care interventions are a net balance between non-maleficence and beneficence. Most treatments carry a risk of some harm; some carry a certainty of harm. Surgical removal of wisdom teeth almost certainly results in pain and swelling, and carries a risk of nerve damage. The net balance for good may be obvious in the face of recurring pericoronitis. The decision to go ahead and have surgery is the patient's, who must balance the risks and benefits and exercise their autonomy following an explanation of risks and benefits.

The same principles apply to the request for a gold crown on an anterior tooth, despite there being no clinical need. There are risks. There are benefits as perceived by the patient, although not by the dentist. Following a *full explanation* of the risks, and certainty that the patient understands those risks, then it is a question of the patient exercising their autonomy. This is the basis of any cosmetic surgery—face lifts, breast and penis enlargement, provision of crowns/veneers to 'straighten crooked teeth' are but a few examples of treatment for which there is no clinical need. The provision of a gold crown, in answer to Kylie's request, therefore seems to fall into that category.

Radiographs of Kylie's teeth are taken. Bitewings, and periapicals UR2, UR1, UL1, UL2, and LL6 show a periapical radiolucency on the mesial root of LL6.

Kylie is pregnant. There are no regulations or even specific guidelines which suggest that dental radiographs should be avoided in pregnant women. However, most dentists would probably limit radiography to the minimum until the pregnancy was over. It could be argued that it was definitely clinically necessary to radiograph Kylie's LL6, as it would not be possible to come to a definitive diagnosis, or make a rational treatment plan, without the information contained in the radiograph. However, the bitewing radiographs and periapicals could have been left untaken until Kylie's baby was born. If Kylie were not pregnant, the choice of radiographs described is appropriate.

A periapical radiolucency on the root of LL6 implies that pulpal necrosis has occurred and that damage has extended to the periapical region, i.e. that the tooth is non-vital. However, very occasionally, in multi-rooted teeth, the pulpal necrosis can occur in relation to one root whilst other parts of the pulp demonstrate some vitality (i.e. the tooth continues to be sensitive to hot, cold, and air drying). Normally, in single-rooted teeth, if there is a periapical radiolucency the tooth is non-vital and will not react to stimuli. Only periapical pressure will cause pain.

Diagnosis

High caries rate with:

1. Mesial and distal caries LR2, LR1, LL1, LL2.
2. Periradicular periodontitis mesial root LL6.
3. Poor appearance UR1, UL1, UL2.

The most pressing concern from the dentist's point of view is to relieve Kylie's pain, although this is not necessarily Kylie's priority. The dentist considers removing the amalgam and placing a sedative dressing. But instead, he opts to extract the tooth at a future visit. Kylie agrees to this course of action.

The question is whether or not Kylie has given an 'informed consent' to the removal of the lower left first molar ('LL6'). It seems that the dentist has considered a sedative dressing but that his decision to extract LL6 is a unilateral one.

A dentist's moral and professional obligations are clear in respect of fully advising a patient in order to help them arrive at a treatment decision. The patient ought to be advised of all the alternatives, the merits of each treatment, the risks of each treatment, the costs of each treatment, and the possible consequences of no treatment. On that basis the patient is able to make an 'informed choice'. The phrase 'informed choice' is preferable to 'informed consent' because there is always a choice of treatments available, even if one of them may be no treatment at all.

Although there can be no doubt that Kylie has consented to the extraction of LL6, in so far as any allegation of assault (more correctly called a battery) is concerned, it is extremely doubtful that in the scenario described, the dentist has fulfilled his professional, moral, and legal duty to furnish Kylie with sufficient information to decide upon the extraction of LL6. In such circumstances, if Kylie could show that had she received proper and adequate advice that she would have opted for a treatment other than extraction then the dentist will be liable for the loss of LL6.

The dentist has done nothing at this visit to relieve Kylie of any pain. He has diagnosed an irreversible pulpitis. However, the dentist's decision to extract the tooth at a future date, rather than dress the tooth now, *may* have been guided by the fact that, in 1997, the Committee on Toxicity of Chemicals in Food, Consumer Products and the Environment concluded that, although there was no evidence to indicate that the placement or removal of dental amalgam fillings during pregnancy is harmful, it is prudent to avoid, where clinically reasonable, the placement or removal of amalgam fillings during pregnancy. The Committee drew this conclusion because the toxicological or epidemiological data were inadequate to fully assess the likelihood of harm arising if fillings were placed or removed during pregnancy, i.e. there was no evidence of harm, but insufficient evidence of 'no harm'.

The dentist explains that Kylie will then need to return for restoration of the lower anterior teeth after the LL6 has been extracted and after that, perhaps, for a crown on UL1 to improve appearance. The dentist does not mention the gold crown for UR2. He does, however, try to explain the process for making and fitting crowns, but Kylie waves his explanations aside, saying she 'knows how it's done, she's had them before'.

The dentist clearly recognizes his professional, moral, and legal obligations to explain treatments to his patients. He has chosen to do so in respect of the provision of a crown at the UL1. However, his explanations of what is involved are brushed aside by Kylie. Thus a question remains: is a patient's decision to have a crown following such a conversation based on adequate information?

This is a matter of autonomy. In many complex issues in health care, a right not to know exists, e.g. genetic testing for hereditary disease. In such cases, parents can choose not to know the results of a genetic test. In that, however, one person's right not to know may be overriden by another person's right to know.

However, in this case Kylie says she knows what is involved. She has already had crowns fitted so it would be reasonable for the dentist to take her word that she fully understands the procedures involved. He cannot force information upon her. The danger is that if something went wrong with the crown then Kylie, being the sort of feisty person she is described as, may wish to complain saying 'I didn't know that my tooth was going to be ground away. The dentist didn't tell me that'. Such a complaint would of course have more substance if Kylie had not had a crown before. Good record keeping is essential, a careful and contemporaneous note of Kylie's waiver is vital.

Second visit: Kylie attends for her extraction. She says the tooth has been worse since the last visit and has woken her up in the night on three occasions.

Toothache which wakens a patient is typical when the pulp is inflamed. This worsening at night has two possible explanations. When a person lies down the blood pressure in the head, and therefore in the teeth, is increased. If a pulp is inflamed, as the blood pressure rises the degree of pain will increase.

Secondly, it may also be the case that toothache which occurs in the day is not as noticeable to the individual concerned while they are busy but becomes unbearable when there is nothing to distract their attention, i.e. when they are asleep or trying to sleep.

Kylie says she has had to take strong painkillers in order to cope with the pain of the toothache.

Kylie is not anxious or nervous about either injection or extractions so the dentist proceeds in the normal way. Two minutes after the administration of the inferior alveolar block, Kylie reports that both her lip and tongue are numb on the left-hand side. The block is supplemented with a long buccal nerve injection. Anaesthesia is checked by probing round the tooth, then the socket expanded using an elevator. Kylie appears to be quite happy and comfortable during these processes.

Finally the forceps are placed on the tooth and the dentist proceeds to extract the tooth.

Pain is best understood as a subjective experience. It does not help the management of the patient to reject the patient's description of their pain. It is the inability of the clinician to have a simultaneous shared experience of the patient's pain that makes it important to listen carefully to the patient's expression of their pain experience. Pain has been defined by the International Association for the Study of Pain (IASP) as 'an unpleasant sensory and emotional experience associated with actual or potential tissue damage or described in terms of such damage'. The definition is helpful as it encourages a view that pain is an emotional experience and not simply a simple direct expression of an extreme sensation. It does differ from other affective states such as anxiety in that pain is focused on some body part, or a part that was present (i.e. 'phantom limb' pain). It is no surprise, therefore, that a relationship between anxiety and pain is shown in various studies, especially when patients are asked to state the pain that they expect to experience from some dental procedure and their dental anxiety. In a major 5-year longitudinal Canadian survey of pain associated with dental treatment, 43% of a sample of over 1400 patients reported having pain during treatment. The number of types of invasive dentistry (e.g. extractions, restoration, etc.) that the patient had received was strongly associated with whether pain had been experienced during the 5-year period under study. Dental attenders who reported pain were more likely to have had a previous painful experience at the dentist, were more dentally anxious, expected dental treatment to be painful, and felt they had little control over the treatment process. When comparisons are made of patients experiences of pain when undergoing pulpectomy or extractions, it is with the latter procedure that patients report significantly higher levels of pain. Hence Kylie's reaction cannot be dismissed or ignored as an exaggerated response. It is likely that past history, expectations, and anxiety are implicated.

The longitudinal study mentioned previously also studied the factors responsible for the development of high levels of dental anxiety. Patients who became dentally anxious over the 5 years of the study were more likely to have experienced pain during dental treatment, more likely to have been treated by a dentist who had an uncaring manner, and more likely to have been frightened or worried about what the dentist did.

The dentist in Kylie's case may have attempted not to present in a cold manner; however, it is important to understand that a patient's perception of the dentist may be related to their general experiences of relating to people. For example, the patient may have great difficulties in establishing a trusting relationship due to poor early family nurturing. The patient may be vulnerable, therefore, to misinterpreting the actions of others. Adults, as well as children, can develop strong dental anxiety responses and this development may be due to a traumatic dental experience and some pre-existing psychological state.

For lower molars, forceps with beaked blades which grip the bifurcation can be used. Alternatively, root pattern forceps gripping the mesial root of the tooth can be used. In difficult lower molar extractions 'cowhorn' forceps, which grip the tooth around the bifurcation, may be useful.

When extracting lower teeth support for the jaw must be given, and the lips, cheeks, and tongue retracted to give maximum visibility. Some operators like to apply a Coupland's elevator mesially and distally to commence movement of the tooth.

Protection of the alveolus is essential prior to guiding the forceps beaks or an elevator on to the tooth. Firm alternating buccal and lingual movements with the forceps, with most pressure being exerted buccally, will usually loosen the tooth. If the buccal bone is very thick, more lingual movement may be necessary. As the tooth becomes loose, mesial rotation of the tooth will assist delivery. If the roots are divergent, or the mandibular bone extremely dense, figure-of-eight movements may be necessary.

Suddenly Kylie shrieks for the dentist to stop. She is crying and says that it hurts 'like hell', as she puts it. The dentist explains patiently that if her tongue, lip, and gums are numb she cannot possibly feel pain from the extraction.

If pain were a purely biological or physiological phenomenon then no-one would experience pain when no injury had occurred and every injury would result in pain. There are thousands of examples which demonstrate that this is not the case—athletes can sustain serious injuries yet do not notice pain until after the competition, amputees often suffer pain from the leg or arm which has been removed, and soldiers with severe injuries may report minimal pain. Thus, it is clear that a person's experience of pain is not simply explained by nerve signals from an injury, but the experience also depends on that person's emotional and evaluative response to the sensations they feel. The end result, the subjective sensation, is as intense as it is felt. No other person can or could possibly decide how much pain another is experiencing, nor could they decree how much pain another person can or should cope with.

Pain is a personal and subjective experience, and the experience of pain will be influenced by both psychological and situational factors. Thus, the amount of pain felt cannot be predicted either from the stimulus or from the amount of anaesthesia or analgesia given.

Kylie feels pain, even though, according to the dentist's knowledge of pharmacology, anatomy, and physiology, she should not have any such sensation. By ignoring Kylie's subjective feelings the dentist is, in effect, saying that those feelings, and Kylie's interpretations of the sensations, are less important than his knowledge. It could be argued that to do this is to cease to regard patients as sentient beings and instead regard them as purely a set of complex anatomical and physiological problems.

If Kylie's dentist had accepted that she was feeling pain, he could have taken steps to reduce, remove, or prevent it.

The dentist tells her that if she did not feel the elevator then the tooth is anaesthetized and that all she is feeling is pressure. After a while, Kylie settles down and appears to have accepted the dentist's interpretation of the situation.

It has already been described that pre-existing psychological difficulties in the patient, the experience of perceived pain, the interpretation of the manner of the dentist, and a sense of reduced control in the operative stage of the dental visit may all have contributed to the intense response of the patient to the loss of their tooth. It is possible to speculate on some plausible alternatives or additional features to help explain the patient's response. It is known that the loss of a tooth can have strong negative associations for patients. In this case Kylie was concerned that losing her tooth in this way would reinforce the view that she is aging. Moreover, she may have been bothered about a change in appearance due to tooth loss. Alternatively, the suggestion floated in the dentist's mind that the patient may have suffered from some physical abuse by her partner, which would also help to explain the conflict raised in the patient when confronted with a potential traumatic episode of an extraction. The patient may feel this, even though the clinical situation of having the tooth extraction is clearly independent of home life. With a high level of anxiety during the preparation of the extraction and during the actual procedure itself the ability of the patient to process logically what is happening to her is reduced.

Once again, the forceps are placed on the tooth and the extraction attempted. Once more, just as the tooth moves significantly in the socket, Kylie yells. This time, she pushes the dentist away and leaps to her feet. She shouts that the dentist is a dangerous and incompetent man, and runs out of the door.

It seems that when Kylie attended for her extraction no further discussion ensued regarding other treatment options. This was the dentist's final chance to discuss other treatment options, and it seems that he did not take it. Even if there had been a full discussion at Kylie's first appointment, when she agreed to extraction it would be vitally important to revisit such a discussion before the extraction commenced.

Adequate anaesthesia appears to have been achieved, but when pressure is put on the tooth with the forceps Kylie experiences great pain. There was no such pain when the socket was being expanded with the elevator. The dentist's attitude is that if her tongue and lip are numb she cannot possibly be feeling any pain from the extraction, but that is not Kylie's perspective!

Legally, once Kylie has pushed the dentist away, her consent for the extraction is withdrawn. That is her choice even though the extraction is incomplete. But her choice results from the dentist's belief and insistence that she was numb. The dentist's failure to investigate Kylie's pain, or improve the anaesthesias, have resulted in Kylie being forced to compromise her own health. In those circumstances the dentist has failed in his professional and moral obligations. The dentist's legal position is also precarious and he would be legally liable for any untoward consequences, which would include the protracted pain of the aborted extraction.

Inexplicable pain during extraction of lower molars, particularly of teeth with long-standing infection, sometimes occurs once significant movement of the tooth is achieved. The problem is best dealt with by adding an infra-ligamentary local anaesthetic to those already given. If anaesthesia is still not achieved then further blocks and infiltration anaesthesia can be tried. If the patient still cannot tolerate the procedure they will have to be admitted to hospital for a general anaesthetic extraction. However, patience and judicious use of local anaesthetic is almost always effective, and extractions rarely fail because of patient's inability to tolerate pain. The maximum adult dose of lidocaine with 1:80 000 epinephrine (adrenaline) is 500 mg.

Five weeks later, Kylie presents at a second dentist. She presents looking completely terrified and asking/begging to see a female dentist. She says that her boyfriend will pay privately for any treatment she has.

Kylie's boyfriend has possibly offered to pay for private treatment because he feels guilty. However, the dentist cannot know this for sure and should not assume it. In fact, the dentist doesn't know whether the boyfriend has offered to pay at all.

Any agreement to provide treatment on a private basis is an agreement between Kylie and the dentist. It is a contract. In general, a contract cannot impose any obligation upon any person who is not a party to it. In these circumstances, Kylie's boyfriend can hardly be described as a party to the contract. He is not even there to agree the price. It would therefore be unfair to impose upon him any legal obligation to pay for Kylie's treatment without any certainty that he is prepared to accept such an obligation. The law of contract is, however, very complex. If the dentist proceeded with treatment and the boyfriend did not pay, as promised by Kylie, then the dentist would have no legal recourse against the boyfriend. It is Kylie who entered in to the contract for private treatment. So, it would be she who would be responsible for any debt due under it.

The situation would be different if the boyfriend was present and he agreed with the dentist in person to pay the cost of Kylie's treatment. This would be a verbal contract for what might not be a very large sum of money. Nevertheless, it is always prudent to put into writing any treatment proposed and its cost. That way, no-one is in any doubt as to what was agreed. It does not require a long or legally drafted contract. A simple letter, setting out what is to be done and its cost, duplicated for a signed returned copy, will suffice.

Kylie has come to the surgery because UR1 has been knocked out, apparently during the course of a domestic dispute. Kylie does not say who was responsible for the injuries to her teeth but the new dentist assumes that it must have been the father of Kylie's unborn child.

Kylie is not saying who was responsible for her injuries, and yet this is a very serious assault. What should the dentist do? If the boyfriend is responsible for Kylie's injuries, there is potential risk to the unborn baby and the possibility that further violence may result in a miscarriage.

However, there is little the dentist can do, or ought to do. Kylie is an adult. If she is the victim of an assault by her boyfriend, or whoever, then she is capable of reporting the matter herself to the police. There is no legal requirement upon anyone to report a crime (save for acts or suspected acts of terrorism). In these circumstances, there is probably no moral obligation, although this could be an arguable position to take. The fact of the pregnancy makes no difference to the dentist's position. Kylie's unborn child has little legal identity, if any, in these circumstances. It is unlikely that Kylie would have any gratitude if the dentist took it upon herself to report the incident. In fact, there may well be professional repercussions for her if she did, as there would be a clear breach of confidentiality.

Clearly as a health-care professional the dentist may have some duty to assist Kylie in dealing with the matter. Some guidance or help to Kylie in seeking further advice would, perhaps, be the very least of the professional obligations the dentist might feel. If such help is rejected then so be it.

As always good record keeping is essential. Kylie might one day report her assailant and the dentist would then be likely to be a witness of fact as to the extent of her injuries.

Domestic violence is not uncommon. In the UK, it is estimated that two women each week are killed by their male partners and other statistics suggest that one in four women are the victims of domestic violence. It occurs in all socioeconomic groups and there is no stereotypical perpetrator. However, a key denominator seems to be an imbalance of power in the relationship. Abuse seems to follow any incident in which the man doubts the respect his partner has for his power. However, they are usually deeply apologetic and emotional after an attack—resulting in the woman forgiving the violence and re-entering the relationship. Gradual erosion of the woman's self-esteem makes it more and more difficult for her to have the strength and courage to leave the relationship. Refuges are available for women suffering domestic violence and in 1999, 54 000 women and children utilized this provision. A national helpline (0800 200 0247) receives approximately 35 000 calls per year from women in violent relationships.

Kylie does not have the avulsed tooth and the incident apparently happened 2 days ago.

Teeth which have been knocked out can sometimes be successfully replanted, i.e. the tooth placed back into its socket under anaesthetic, held in place for 3–4 min, and splinted. However, the prognosis of the tooth depends largely on the amount of time the tooth has been out of the mouth and whether it has been correctly stored or allowed to dry out. Any tooth which has been out of the mouth for more than 2 h is unlikely, if replanted, to reattach, and may undergo external and internal resorption. Replantation in Kylie's case would therefore not be an option.

The female dentist agrees to construct an acrylic denture for Kylie but advises her that, so long as her oral hygiene remains good, other more permanent solutions might be possible. Kylie states that she will not have any treatment other than the denture, as she 'does not trust' dentists.

A longitudinal study of extremely dentally anxious patients within a local authority housing estate found that after attending a number of group sessions the patients were able to visit a community service dentist. It was found that the difference between those who attended regularly and those who attended only when in trouble was related to the dentist remembering to ask the patient how they felt about dental procedures, even some months or years after an initial successful visit. Some patients who decided not to attend regularly had found that dentists had forgotten that they were anxious about dentistry and rushed treatment. Hence it is possible to translate the abstract sense of trust that patients say that they require in a dentist into actions that support or reduce that belief.

However, when the denture is delivered, Kylie is so relieved and pleased with her improved appearance that she becomes a little more relaxed. The dentist takes time to explain that the fit of the denture will change as the gums remodel, and that she will need a new denture, or an alternative, within the near future.

Following dental extractions, there is a reduction in the size of the alveolar ridge. The rate and amount of change varies between patients, but the greatest change occurs in the first 6 months after extraction, with the denture-bearing area becoming stable after 1 year. Remodelling (mainly resorption) of the ridge continues throughout life. An immediate denture will quickly lose its adaptation to the supporting tissues during the first 6 months and may need relining or replacement during that time.

Kylie promises to attend every 6 months after the birth of her child, which is now due in 2 months' time.

At each of Kylie's subsequent visits, Kylie's confidence in the dentist grows but she claims she cannot and will not have any treatment which involves injections or potential pain 'unless she is knocked out'.

Dental anxiety assessment and its clinical implications

Kylie's sense of control over her own life and her own teeth has been minimized by her circumstances and by the things which have happened to her.

Kylie appears to have little control over her domestic situation and over her finances, and has had experiences which would suggest to anyone in Kylie's position that they had little control over what happens either in the dental chair or in their home.

She is therefore bound to have an external locus of control. Expecting, and only accepting, treatment under anaesthesia is the ultimate externalization of control.

What is required is that Kylie starts to feel some sense of control again. This can be encouraged by allowing her to make decisions in the dental surgery (and these decisions being accepted even if the dentist does not wholeheartedly agree with them); by using stop signals, and by listening to Kylie's interpretation of the world.

There are two major approaches within practice that can be recommended for the assessment of the dentally anxious patient. The first is the use of a questionnaire that patients can complete within the waiting room. There are a number of standardized measures that can be used routinely. They have the advantage that they can be stored easily with the patient notes as a reminder on subsequent visits about the patient's anxiety and any particular procedure or event in the surgery that causes particular difficulty. The Dental Fear Schedule is a scale comprising 15 questions. It provides some specific information about the patient's feelings towards the practice, other staff and the dentist. The length of the 15-item measure tends to reduce its use, as not only can patients find it a burden, but also the dentist may have difficulty in quickly summarizing the results from a simple 'eye-balling' of the replies. It is, however, an excellent measure for research projects. Corah's Dental Anxiety Scale (CDAS) contains only four questions and has been used extensively with adult patients in many countries. It has a possible range of scores from a minimum of 4 to a maximum of 20. An arbitrary cut-off of greater than 15 is commonly recognized. An improved measure: the Modified Dental Anxiety Scale (MDAS) consists of five questions similar to the CDAS with the added item of having an injection. The answering scheme has been made consistent across all questions making comparison easy. The extra item enables the dentist to get an opinion from the patient about his/her anxiety about local anaesthesia, which has been found previously to be the most anxiety-provoking procedure. A score of 19 or greater has been shown (using a reference group of dentally anxious patients) to indicate patients with extreme dental anxiety.

The handing of the completed questionnaire by the patient to the dentist in the surgery provides a unique opportunity for the dentist to get a brief overview of the patient's possible reaction to the procedures that the dentist may attempt. Some evidence suggests that the physical handing over of the questionnaire to the dentist assists in some way in reducing the anxiety of patients. Exactly how this anxiety reduction can be explained is not clear at present. The physical delivery by the patient to the dentist of a record of his/her anxiety about a number of dental procedures may enhance the expectations that patients hold about their visit, thinking that the dentist now knows how they feel and therefore believing that the dentist will be even more careful in their treatment. Alternatively the dentist may simply change their clinical approach and attend more closely to the patient's sensitivities about receiving treatment. Of course, in reality, it may be a mixture of both effects.

Patients who score above the dental anxiety cut-off points referred to above require some extra assistance from within the practice, or a referral to specialist treatment services at a local dental hospital should be made.

After 2 years the nurse finally manages to persuade Kylie to have her teeth radiographed and a large periapical radiolucency is visible, associated with UL1. The dentist explains that root treatment is required in order to make sure that symptoms do not arise. Kylie asks: '… if there's a problem, why doesn't it hurt'? When the dentist argues that it *may* hurt in the future, Kylie asks what percentage of teeth like her UL1 start to hurt. In the end Kylie says that she will attend to have the tooth treated if it begins to hurt.

As discussed at several junctures in this book, all clinical treatment should commence with the patient making an informed choice about treatment. This requires that the dentist tell the patient about both the benefits *and* the less positive outcomes which may result from treatment. It is particularly important that dentists are able to address specific questions about outcomes when treatment is to be offered to a patient who is entirely free from symptoms.

Kylie, quite reasonably, is trying, through her questions, to ascertain what benefits she might accrue by having the root treatment which the dentist has suggested. It appears to her, from the dentist's answer, that she is not necessarily going to gain any benefit—she is merely going to reduce the chances of a negative occurrence (pain from the tooth). Whilst it may seem odd to members of the dental profession that the patient does not want to pursue this risk reduction strategy, this behaviour is perfectly in keeping with what is known about individuals' risk attitudes. Generally, people tend to think of small probabilities as larger than they actually are. They also think of large probabilities as being smaller than they actually are. Thus, if the dentist says that the tooth will 'in all probability become painful' or says that 'there's a high chance it will become sore' then Kylie will make a lower estimate of the likelihood of this poor outcome than the dentist has made. In contrast, if a dentist says that 'it's very unlikely' or 'only one in a million' teeth like Kylie's become painful, she is likely to make a higher estimate than the dentist's of the tooth becoming painful.

Furthermore, people's choices are also influenced by how 'bad' they think they will feel about having made a poor decision (i.e. one which leads to poor outcomes). The regret a person will feel if things go wrong immediately after a behaviour is much more powerful than the regret they will feel if they experience poor consequences some time after *not* doing a behaviour. That is, to Kylie, if the tooth becomes painful as a result of her inaction, that's sort of, 'just life'. However, if she has some treatment done on the tooth and she suffers pain as a consequence, this will affect her more and be a cause for great regret about the decision she made.

Hence, her decision is to leave the tooth untreated until pain arises. Should the tooth spontaneously become painful in the future, she will have something done about it at that point. Her reasoning is along the lines of 'if it ain't broke (which to her it is not) don't fix it'. To the dentist, there is a problem with the tooth but he must respect Kylie's personal autonomy and should try to understand her viewpoint.

If one thinks hard about it, treating an asymptomatic tooth 'in case' it causes problems is actually quite illogical—unless the chances of symptoms are extremely high and the consequences of those symptoms are very severe (i.e. the tooth will be agonizing). Thus, it is essential that the dentist is able to inform the patient of both the probability and the severity of sequelae from treatment *and* from non-treatment. In this particular instance, the dentist needs to be able to tell Kylie the answer to her question about the likelihood of pain arising in the tooth, preferably in numerical terms, i.e. Kylie really needs to know the answer to the following: if 100 teeth with periapical radiolucencies which were asymptomatic and not root treated were left untreated, how many would cause problems?

The answer to this question is, unfortunately, unknown. But given the number of periapical radiolucencies observed on non-symptomatic teeth, it would seem likely that the answer to Kylie's question is quite a small percentage. Such gaps in the evidence base are problematic, as truly informed consent is not achievable in the absence of the relevant and appropriate information. However, research continues apace and hopefully, in time, the answers to all questions relevant to clinical dentistry will become available.

Although all patients must give informed consent to treatment, not all will willingly participate in decision-making as Kylie has. Each patient has a preferred decision role. That is, some people prefer the dentist to make the decisions and want the professional to simply inform them of what they think best, whilst others would be most dismayed at such an approach and like to make the decisions themselves. The majority, studies have shown, want a collaborative approach where dentist and patient make any decisions jointly. The problem with this variability in decision-making style is that the dentist needs to vary his/her approach according to the patient's preferred role. This is not always easy.

However, it is vital with all patients to try to move them away from the 'dentist-knows-best-and-will-choose' attitude. This is because people who regard their health problems as 'someone else's' (i.e. the doctor's or the dentist's) are very unlikely to take action on behalf of their own health. This is because they have a core belief that their health is not their responsibility and not under their control, thereby reducing their internal health locus of control. People with an external locus of control are less likely to undertake a good home care regime. Preventive messages are unlikely to be acted on if the patient does not believe they 'own' their oral health. Thus, patient-led, or at least shared decision-making is preferable, not least because it helps to engender a belief of personal commitment to healthiness by the patient.

A further 2 years later Kylie attends again, with her 4-year-old child. She has been experiencing problems with the UL1, but is still extremely fearful of treatment. She explains that this is so because of the dentist who hurt her, nearly 5 years ago. She explains how she had to go to hospital to have the tooth which he had loosened taken out under general anaesthetic, but that the experience with the dentist, who would not take any notice of her screams, was the worst thing that ever happened to her, and that she now cannot ever trust anyone to put any sort of instrument in her mouth.

A phobia is 'a compelling fear or dread, especially of a particular object or situation'. Thus, dentists actually very rarely see people who are truly phobic. A true dental phobic is 'compelled' to avoid dentistry at all costs, will endure unbelievable pain, and will demonstrate physiological signs of pain and anxiety if they enter a surgery, or, in some people, even talk about dentistry.

Thus, the vast majority of people who are labelled 'phobic' of dentistry, or 'needle phobic' are in fact, not suffering from a phobia. They may be very anxious, or fearful, or worried but they are not 'phobic'. Kylie is very frightened of having pain inflicted on her by someone she ought to be able to trust. Although this is a very difficult type of patient to deal with, it is neither correct, necessary, nor helpful to label them as having a phobia.

The dentist then offers treatment to Kylie under inhalation sedation, explains that no injections will be needed, and talks to Kylie about stop signals.

Inhalation sedation is a method used along with adjunctive cognitive behavioural procedures and hypnotic suggestion. The combination of approaches applied by a sensitive clinician can greatly assist patients, particularly those who are very anxious. The patient's coping mechanisms are enhanced and encouraged to foster a relaxed state during dental treatment. It is an extremely safe technique, which is suitable for use with both adults and children. It cannot be over-emphasized that the effectiveness of inhalation sedation is hugely dependent on the behavioural management skills of the operator.

The patient undergoing treatment breathes, through a small nose piece, a mixture of oxygen and nitrous oxide. The amount of each gas is titrated against the patient's needs and is therefore dependent on the patient's initial level of anxiety and upon the procedure which is to be undertaken. Typically, 25–30% nitrous oxide gives good sedation but this is very variable. Some patients may be deeply sedated breathing 10–15% whilst others will require >40% nitrous oxide. The key is to treat each patient as an individual and to be very aware of the patient's level of relaxation.

Adequately sedated patients respond slowly to questions, stare into the middle distance, seem calm and happy, and show no sign of muscle tension.

Care must be taken not to over-sedate patients, as doing so can turn a pleasant experience for the patient into an unpleasant one. An appropriately sedated patient will report that they felt warm and euphoric. Some will say that they experienced a tingling sensation, some will feel light, some heavy, some as if they are floating. Like the 'correct' level of nitrous oxide, the sensations felt by sedated patients are extremely variable.

Inhalation sedation is an extremely useful and, perhaps, under-utilized technique. Most importantly, it is amazingly safe. In over 50 years of use, there have not been any reports of mortality or serious morbidity associated with it.

In Kylie's case, inhalation sedation would seem to be an ideal approach in order to try to reduce her anxiety and build her confidence in dentists and dentistry. Also, because the tooth to be treated is known to be non-vital, no local anaesthesia will be required and therefore the whole treatment experience will hopefully be a positive one.

One particularly important technique to use with patients who have had, but lost, confidence in dentistry is stop signals. These, as explained in an earlier chapter, are signs or movements which the patient and dentist agree will stop the dentistry proceeding. Thus, Kylie should be told that the dentist will always stop what is being done if she (for example) waves her right hand.

Kylie has clearly developed a very 'external' locus of control in relation to dentistry. She feels (understandably) that she, the patient, has no 'say' or control over what happens to her. Her preference is to be as passive a patient as it is possible to be, i.e. unconscious under anaesthesia. If Kylie's confidence is to be built, she needs to recognize that she can control proceedings. Stop signals are also a very useful technique to employ with child patients. The only proviso about the use of stop signals is, for some patients, that the responsibility to indicate when they wish to stop can become overwhelming. That is, the patient can become anxious about interrupting the dentist's work and believe that some danger may befall themselves. For example, the patient may consider that stopping the dentist in the middle of drilling may put the dentist off and therefore force the dentist to make an error and spoil the tooth, or worse might send the drill on an erratic course into the patient's cheek and cause injury. Catastrophic thinking is common in anxious patients. To prevent this scenario, the dentist would need to ensure that their explanation to the patient included a reassurance that the procedure could be safely stopped at any time. Once this explanation has been given, the patient is asked if they would like to practise the procedure and the patient is invited to deliberately stop the dentist even if the patient can tolerate the procedure easily. The dentist should remember to praise the patient for their perseverance and good progress. Therefore, a repetitive reminder that the patient is doing well is recommended. Best practice would be demonstrated by the dentist acknowledging the patient's forbearance on occasions when the dentist makes a change of drill bit, alters postural position, or stops the procedure to examine carefully the technical success of the treatment.

In summary, the dentist promises the patient, at the outset, that if anything is troubling them, or they simply want a rest, all they have to do is make a particular signal (usually using the right hand) and the dentist will stop.

The dentist must be scrupulous about always obeying the stop signal.

With or without the practice procedures in trying out the use of stop signals, the patient may use the approach once or twice near the beginning of the treatment to 'test' that it 'works'. Many patients, once they realize that they have reliable control over the process, relax completely.

After a number of acclimatization visits, at which Kylie is slowly introduced to treatment, Kylie copes well with the root canal treatment of UL1. Having gained some confidence she then requests that you place a gold crown on this tooth. She also says that the denture carrying UR1 is causing her great embarrassment when she sings, as it drops down sometimes.

There is not a simple one-to-one relationship between symptoms or signs of disease and a person's own rating of quality of life. The term quality of life may be defined as 'when the hopes of an individual are met and fulfilled by experience'. The link between the hopes of a patient being achieved and their symptom experience may be tenuous at best. The definition supplied here is based on the wants of the individual being satisfied. However, this is one of many definitions. Various measures of general quality of life have been developed (e.g. the Short Form 36 and Sickness Impact Profile) which are relatively short questionnaires which patients complete themselves.

Quality of life by definition is subjective and the clinician's rating is frequently at odds with the patient-derived estimate. To improve responsiveness it is common for clinicians and researchers alike to adopt patient-completed health-related measures of quality of life specific to the condition under investigation. For oral health problems there are now a variety of measures available, including, for instance, the Oral Health–Quality of Life UK (OH–QoL UK), Oral Health Impact Profile (OHIP), General Oral Health Assessment Scales (GOHAI), and the Subjective Oral Health Status Indicators (SOHSI). All of them produce summary scores for various domains of function or psychosocial consequences. For example, the Dental Impact Profile (DIP) assesses four subscales derived from 25 questions, namely eating, health/well-being, social relations, and romance. The patient is asked to rate from positive to negative various statements such as: 'do you think your teeth or dentures have a good effect, a bad effect or no effect on your eating?'. An overall score can also be simply calculated. The scores derived can be compared against various normative values obtained from different reference groups to help gain an assessment of the relative position of the patient. Profiles of the patient can be compiled over time to establish the change in oral health quality of life. Other factors can be introduced to assist in assessing the influence of the oral condition on the patient's overall well-being taking in account their current life circumstances. Kylie, for instance, will probably rate her oral health quality of life as deficient in the area of social relations. Careful questioning by the dentist of course could encourage these concerns to be discussed, but using measures of this type can establish efficiently where a patient's concerns really lie. It is known from a large representative UK survey that regular attenders to the dentist tend to rate their oral health-related quality of life more positively, whereas those who are dentally anxious are among those with the poorest ratings of life quality. However, slavish adherence to these measures is not recommended, and from a clinical perspective they may be employed simply as a device to encourage a more comprehensive assessment in discussion with the patient.

Treatment options

Kylie has a reasonably intact but heavily restored dentition and has UR1 missing. UL1 is root filled and heavily restored, UL2 is crowned, UR2 is sound.

The options to replace UR1 that should be discussed with Kylie are:

- Another denture—in either acrylic or cobalt chrome: This is the most retrievable situation as no or minimal tooth preparation would be required. Dentures can also replace bone and soft tissue as well as teeth, and if there had been significant resorption then this may be a good option. However, the risks of partial dentures include increased plaque and caries levels and increased numbers of root surface restorations. Kylie has managed to wear the partial denture, which was fitted immediately following the loss of the tooth, and there will have been bone resorption since that time resulting in loss of stability and retention of the denture. If she were provided with a better-fitting and more retentive denture then she may cope quite well.

- Resin-retained bridge: If the UL1 were sound and the occlusion favourable this would be a strong contender for restoring the UR1 space. However, the large restorations in the UL1 would be difficult to replace or repair if they failed when a resin-retained bridge was in place.

- Conventional bridge: When there are heavily restored teeth adjacent to the missing tooth/teeth, then a conventional bridge becomes a likely option. In Kylie's case it may be possible to cantilever the UR1 pontic from a retainer on the UL1.

- Implant: An implant would be possible in this situation although if Kylie still smokes this may be considered a contraindication to implant provision. Other concerns are the long-term prognosis for Kylie's remaining upper anterior teeth, as the UL1 and UL2 are heavily restored and UL1 is root filled.

Kylie opts for an acrylic denture as she feels this will suit her best and she can always go for another of the options at a later date. The dentist suggests to Kylie that she bring her daughter along with her when she comes for her appointments.

Parents of young children, although they may themselves be resistant to changing their own health-related behaviours, are often very open to advice regarding their children. Thus, if a patient has children it is often worthwhile explaining the principles of preventing dental disease in the context of preventing disease in the patient's child. Very often, because both diet and brushing are so intimately bound up with a person's general home life, any behaviours which are introduced for the benefit of young children may spread to other members of the family, even the adults and parents.

BIBLIOGRAPHY

Allen PF. Assessment of oral health related quality of life. *Health and Quality of Life Outcomes 2003*, 1:40 (http://www.hqlo.com/content/1/1/40)

Anderson R, Thomas DW. 'Toothache stories': a qualitative investigation of why and how people seek emergency dental care. *Community Dental Health* 2003; **20**: 106–111.

Andreasen J. *Essentials of Traumatic Injuries to the Teeth*, 2nd edn. Munksgaard: Copenhagen, 2000.

Bandolier: Evidence-based thinking about health care. www.jr2.ox.ac.uk/bandolier

Berggren U, Pierce CJ, Eli I. Characteristics of adult dentally fearful individuals. A cross-cultural study. *European Journal of Oral Science* 2000; **108**: 268–274.

Blain KM, Hill F. The use of inhalation sedation and local anaesthesia as an alternative to general anaesthesia for dental extractions in children. *British Dental Journal* 1998; **184**: 608–611.

Blinkhorn AS, Mackie IC. *Practical Treatment Planning for the Paedodontic Patient*. Quintessence: London, 1997.

British National Formulary. British Medical Association and Royal Pharmaceutical Society of Great Britain: London, 2004.

Callum C. *The UK Smoking Epidemic: Deaths in 1995*. HEA: London, 1998.

Chapple H, Shah S, Caress AL, Kay EJ. Exploring dental patients preferred roles in treatment decision-making—a novel approach. *British Dental Journal* 2003; **194**: 321–327.

Chestnutt IG, Binnie VI. Smoking cessation counselling—a role for the dental profession. *British Dental Journal* 1995; **179**: 411–415.

Cohen SM, Fiske J, Newton JT. The impact of dental anxiety on daily living. *British Dental Journal* 2000; **189**: 385–390.

Dailey Y-M, Crawford AN, Humphris GM, Lennon MA. Long term effects on dental anxiety, dental beliefs and dental attendance behaviour, following anxiety treatment in a primary care setting. *Primary Dental Care* 2001; **8**(2): 19–24.

Dailey YM, Humphris GM, Lennon MA. Reducing dental patient's state anxiety in general dental practice. A randomised controlled trial. *Journal of Dental Research* 2002; **81**(5): 319–322.

Eli I, Uziel N, Baht R, Kleinhauz M. Antecedents of dental anxiety: learned responses versus personality traits. *Community Dentistry and Oral Epidemiology* 1997; **25**: 233–237.

Feinmann, C. *The Mouth, the Face and the Mind*. Oxford University Press: Oxford, 1999.

Freeman R. A psychodynamic theory for dental phobia. *British Dental Journal* 1998; **184**: 170–172.

Hagglin C, Hakeberg M, Ahlquist M, Sullivan M, Berggren U. Factors associated with dental anxiety and attendance in middle aged and elderly women. *Community Dentistry and Oral Epidemiology* 1999; **28**: 451–460.

Humphris GM, Ling MS. *Behavioural Sciences for Dentistry*. Churchill Livingstone: Edinburgh, 2000.

Humphris GM, Morrison T, Lindsay SJE. The Modified Dental Anxiety Scale: validation and United Kingdom norms. *Community Dental Health* 1995; **12**: 143–150.

Ingersoll BD. *Behavioural Aspects in Dentistry*. Appleton-Century-Crofts: New York, 1982.

Johnson NW, Bain C. Tobacco and oral disease. *British Dental Journal* 2000; **4**: 200–206.

Kay EJ, Blinkhorn AS. A qualitative investigation of factors governing dentists' treatment philosophies. *British Dental Journal* 1996; **180**: 171–176.

Kay EJ, Nuttall NM. Assessing risks and probabilities. *British Dental Journal* 1995; **178**: 153–155.

Kay EJ, Nuttall NM. Patient preferences and their influence on decision making. *British Dental Journal* 1995; **178**: 229–233.

Kay EJ, Tinsley S. *Communication for the Dental Team*. Partners in Practice: Northants, 1995.

Lindsay SJ, Roberts GJ, Wardle J, Woolgrove J, Yates J. Fear and pain in routine dentistry. *British Dental Journal* 1982; **152**: 3–4.

Locker D, Shapiro D, Liddell A. Negative dental experiences and their relationship to dental anxiety. *Community Dental Health* 1996; **13**: 86–92.

Maggirias J, Locker D. Psychological factors and perceptions of pain associated with dental treatment. *Community Dentistry and Oral Epidemiology* 2002; **30**(2): 151–159.

Matthews R, Zakrewska JM, Harrison SD (eds). *Assessment and Management of Orofacial Pain*. Elsevier: London, 2002.

McGrath C, Bedi R. Dental attendance, oral health and the quality of life. *British Dental Journal* 2001; **190**: 262–265.

National Health Service Executive. *Patient Partnership: Building a Collaborative Strategy*. Department of Health: London, 1996.

Newton JT, Buck DJ. Anxiety and pain measures in dentistry: a guide to their quality and application. *Journal of the American Dental Association* 2000; **131**(10): 1449–1457.

Pau AKH, Croucher R, Marcenes N. Perceived inability to cope and care seeking in patients with toothache: a qualitative study. *British Dental Journal* 2000; **189**: 503–506.

Roberts GJ. Inhalation sedation with oxygen/nitrous oxide gas. *Dental Update* 1990; **17**: 190–196.

Roberts GJ, Brook AH, Page J, Davenport EJ. A policy document for inhalation sedation. *International Journal of Paediatric Dentistry* 1996; **6**: 63–66.

Rotter JB. *Social Learning and Clinical Psychology*. Prentice Hall: Englewood Cliffs, NJ, 1954.

Rotter JB. Some problems and misconceptions related to the construct of internal versus external control of reinforcement. *Journal of Consulting and Clinical Psychology* 1975; **43**: 56–67.

Rotter JB, Chance J, Phares EJ (eds). *Applications of a Social Learning Theory of Personality*. Holt, Rinehart and Winston: New York, 1972.

Selection Criteria for Dental Radiography. Faculty of General Dental Practitioners: London, 2004.

Shaw AJ, Meechan JG, Kilpatrick NM, Welbury R. The use of inhalation sedation and local anaesthesia for extraction and minor oral surgery in children. *International Journal of Paediatric Dentistry* 1996; **6**: 7–11.

Smith SE, Warnakulasuriya KAAS, Feyerabend C, Belcher M, Cooper DJ, Johnson NW. A smoking cessation programme conducted through dental practices in the UK. *British Dental Journal* 1998; **185**: 299–303.

Smoking Kills: a White Paper on Tobacco. The Stationery Office: London, 1998.

Sondell K, Söderfeldt B, Palmqvist S. Underlying dimensions of verbal communication between dentists and patients in prosthetic dentistry. *Patient Education and Counselling* 2003; **50**: 157–165.

Thomson WM, Locker D, Poulton R. Incidence of dental anxiety in young adults in relation to dental treatment experience. *Community Dentistry and Oral Epidemiology* 2000; **28**: 289–294.

Wallston KA, Wallston BS, DeVellis R. Development of the multidimensional health locus of control scales. *Health Education Monographs* 1978; **6**: 160–170.

Watt R, Robinson M. *Helping Smokers to Stop—a Guide for the Dental Team.* HEA: London, 1999.

Watt RG, Daly B, Kay EJ. Smoking cessation advice within the general dental practice. *British Dental Journal* 2003; **194**: 665–668.

Wilks C. Dental phobia. *British Dental Journal* 1998; **185**: 266.

Robert is a 9-year-old lad who lives in a village. It is a quiet and friendly village with a pub, a post office, and a village green. The village's only dental practice is situated near to the doctor's surgery on a corner of the green. On summer evenings and through the holidays Robert and his friend Jaz like to play either football or cricket on the green with their friends. Robert is a 'ringleader' in the activities and is the one who organizes the children into teams so that they can play impromptu matches.

Robert had been attending the village's dental practice since his first tooth erupted but had never needed any treatment, other than the dentist keeping a watchful eye on Robert's quite severe Class II division 1 malocclusion.

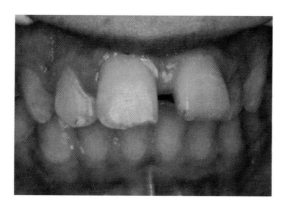

Class II division 1 malocclusion

Why are Class II/1 malocclusions of concern to dentists (other than because of aesthetics)?

Why has the dentist not treated Robert's malocclusion and how should this be done?

One evening, the dentist and his nurse were just saying goodbye to the last patient, sorting out the surgery, and planning to leave when Robert came running into the waiting room. Robert was followed by his mate, Jaz, who was carrying a tooth. Robert was white and looked very shaken and was holding his hands over his mouth.

'I got hit', he mumbled to the dentist through his hands, 'with the bat, the cricket bat'. The dentist's nurse ushered Robert into the surgery and got him to sit on the dental chair. She retrieved the tooth from Jaz, who had been alert enough to spot the tooth in the grass, wrap it in his handkerchief and run with Robert to the surgery. She washed it gently and popped the tooth into a bowl of saline.

Should this tooth be replanted?

The dentist asked Jaz, who was aged 8, what had happened. Jaz said that there had been an argument amongst the boys about whether Robert, who had been keeping wicket, had stumped Zachary Brown out. Zac had got cross, explained Jaz, when Rob said he was out, then Zac swung the bat and hit Robert round the face.

Why did the dentist ask Jaz what had happened?

The dentist then went to see Robert, who was in the surgery with the nurse. Although he was pale and obviously in pain, he did not seem overly upset.

What was Robert's reaction to the trauma?

'Okay Rob', the dentist asked, 'what happened?'

'Oh, I was wicket keeping and he went to take a huge shot. I was too close, and got hit.'

The dentist ascertained from Robert that there had been little delay in coming to the surgery, although Robert said he had fallen to the floor and wasn't sure how long he had lain there. The dentist checked with Jaz, who said that Robert had got straight up. The dentist tried to find out who else had been there but Rob seemed a bit vague about the answer to this question.

Why did the dentist ask how long it had taken the children to get to the surgery?
What should the dentist do first?

Given that Robert seemed not to be too badly hurt, the dentist then suggested that he examine his teeth whilst the nurse tried to ring Robert's mother. The dentist knew that although Robert's father still lived in the village, he was divorced from Robert's mother.

'She's not in', said Rob. 'She's gone to the supermarket. She'll be about an hour and a half.'

'Well, who's looking after you?' asked the nurse.

'I hate going to the supermarket so mum always says that I can stay and play on the green 'til she gets back.'

The nurse then thought to ask:

'Where's your dad then?'

'Dunno', was the reply, 'but my gran's number is 0483.'

The dentist decided that he would go ahead and examine Robert's mouth anyway and Robert seemed happy about this.

Rob's lower lip was bruised and swollen with two small lacerations on the oral surface. He had a graze on his chin and his left cheek.

What should the dentist do about Robert's injuries?

The upper right central incisor was missing—presumably the tooth which Jaz had been carrying which was now residing in the bowl of saline. The upper

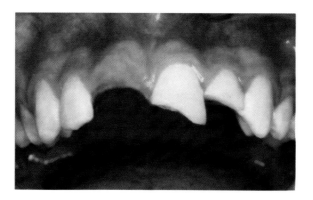

Fractured incisors and missing UR1

right lateral incisor was extremely mobile and had been displaced palatally. Its position meant that Robert could not close his back teeth together. The upper left central incisor was fractured. The fracture ran from the mesial edge, almost at the gingival level, to the disto-incisal corner through enamel denture and pulp. The pulpal exposure was approximately 1 mm in diameter. The upper left lateral incisor had a enamel fracture on the incisal edge.

The dentist told Robert that he could put the tooth back in place, but that he would need to have an injection. Robert was not particularly happy about this, but, having asked questions about whether it would hurt, agreed to try.

How typical was Robert's view of having an injection?

Jaz helped to encourage Robert's decision by saying how he'd had injections at the dentist and that it hadn't hurt. The dentist therefore anaesthetized the UR1 socket, replanted the tooth and aligned the UR2. He also placed calcium hydroxide on the pulpal exposure and the dentine on UL1 and placed a composite bandage on the tooth.

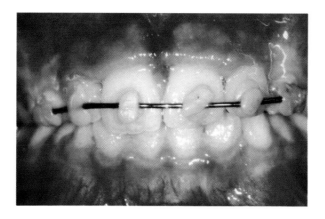

An example of splinting with wire and composite

Why should a composite bandage be placed?

The replanted UR1 and mobile UR2 were splinted to UL1 and UL2. More stable splinting was not possible as neither the canines nor the premolar teeth had yet erupted.

The nurse sat with Jaz who, just as the dentist was finishing the work, pointed and said: 'There's Rob's mum.'

The nurse rushed out on to the green and said: 'I'm afraid Robert has had a little accident'.

Robert's mother blanched and she wobbled on her feet.

'Oh, he's okay, he's okay, it's just his teeth.'

'His teeth', his mum cried. 'His lovely new teeth.'

The nurse ushered Robert's mother towards the dental practice. Just as they came through the main door, Robert and the dentist emerged from the surgery.

Robert's mother hugged Robert and the dentist explained what he had done and what Robert had said had happened. The dentist then took Robert's mother to one side and explained that Jaz's story had been a little different from Robert's. The dentist suggested that she might wish to make further enquiries from Robert's friends.

Robert and his mother then went home, with an appointment to return in a week's time. As it was now quite late in the evening, the dentist thought he would write up Robert's notes the following day.

What advantages are there in writing up notes immediately after seeing the patient?

Later that evening, the dentist became increasingly concerned that he had witnessed the results of a quite vicious assault. He became so worried about this that eventually he telephoned the police and reported what had happened.

The following week, Robert and his mother attended for Robert's appointment. Robert's mum was angry. Firstly, the police had been to her house as a result of the dentist's phone call. She was most distressed that the police had become involved in an incident in which, according to her was 'boys being boys'. Another reason she was annoyed was because, for the last two nights, Robert had been kept awake by intense pain from both of the central incisor teeth.

'I wish you'd never put that tooth back in. It's causing trouble and I know it's going to end up being more trouble than it's worth.'

The dentist tried to explain the reasons he replanted Robert's tooth, to which the mother replied that: 'you should never have done it without my say so'.

The dentist recognized that the teeth were pulpitic, probably irreversibly so. He explained to Robert and his mother that he would need to remove the pulps from the teeth and put something in the teeth to help the root to form.

Why is Robert experiencing pain?
How does treatment help the tooth root to form?

The dentist proceeded to extirpate the central incisors under local anaesthetic, noticing as he did so that although UR2 had firmed up well, UR1 did not appear to be any more stable than when he had just replanted it.

Despite weekly visits, repeated splinting and 3-monthly applications of CaOH to the root canal, UR1 failed to become firm. After 9 months, UR1 was extracted and a single tooth denture provided for Robert.

What type of denture should be made for Robert?

At this point, the calcific barrier at the apex of UL1 was considered well developed. The tooth was root filled.

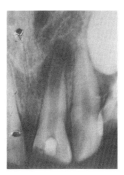 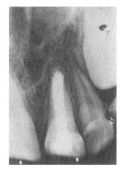

Radiographs of immature
UL1, apexification and RCT

Describe how to root fill an immature incisor.

Robert and his mother then voiced increasing concern about Robert's 'goofy' appearance. Robert said that he is teased at school and called names because of his protruding front teeth.

Is it possible to treat Robert's malocclusion when he already has a denture?

Robert also says that the denture 'looks horrible' and 'made it impossible' for him to play the flute which he had started learning. The dentist therefore referred Robert to an orthodontist.

Fortunately, Robert did not have crowding in either arch and the orthodontist wrote back to the dentist to say that he would treat Robert with a functional appliance.

What could have been done if Robert had had crowding?

The orthodontist thought Robert would cope with the functional appliance and the denture at the same time. However, he also expressed concern that the short root on UL1 may make it more than usually liable to resorption.

Robert continued to have good oral health other than his malocclusion and some problems with the denture. When he was 16, the dentist suggested that

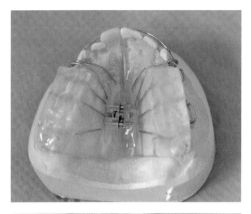

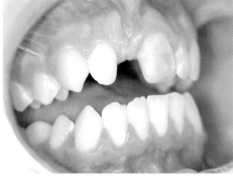

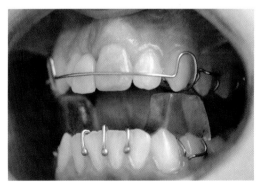

Functional appliance with prosthetic tooth to replace UR1

the denture could be replaced with a resin-retained bridge. This would then be followed, once Robert's jaw has stopped growing, by a single tooth implant. Thus, at aged 21 an implant was placed to replace UR1.

For years, Robert's implant was fine, then, suddenly, aged 27, he noticed that the tooth had become mobile.

Eventually, the decision was made that the implant would have to be removed. The treatment options at this stage were:

- re-implant
- ceramic bridge

- adhesive bridges
- denture.

Robert and the dentist discussed the options. Robert asked his dentist for more information on the relative longevity of each of the options. Eventually, after much discussion, Robert decided that he preferred a bridge to the alternative treatments.

Three weeks later, the dentist started Robert's treatment.

Ten years later, Robert's bridge is intact. He is a regular dental attender and now brings his family along for dental check-ups. Robert is assiduous in the care of his children's teeth, presumably because of the problems his dental injury caused him.

The dentist is careful to offer appropriate advice. This includes encouragement of brushing the children's teeth with a fluoride toothpaste.

Why not offer Robert's children fluoride supplements?

The dentist has also warned Robert about the possibility of his children requiring orthodontic treatment as they get older, as facial growth to some extent follows a familial pattern. Finally, the dentist advises that Robert's children should wear mouthguards when playing contact sports.

Should the dentist make Robert's children wear their mouthguards?

Robert's two children grow up with intact dentitions but both require orthodontic treatment with functional and fixed appliances when they reach their early teenage years.

Why would Robert's children require fixed braces?

ROBERT: A TRAUMATIC BLOW

Robert is a 9-year-old lad who lives in a village. It is a quiet and friendly village with a pub, a post office, and a village green. The village's only dental practice is situated near to the doctor's surgery on a corner of the green. On summer evenings and through the holidays Robert and his friend Jaz like to play either football or cricket on the green with their friends. Robert is a 'ringleader' in the activities and is the one who organizes the children into teams so that they can play impromptu matches.

Robert had been attending the village's dental practice since his first tooth erupted but had never needed any treatment, other than the dentist keeping a watchful eye on Robert's quite severe Class II division 1 malocclusion.

Class II division 1 malocclusions are known to increase the incidence of trauma to the anterior teeth by threefold if the overjet is greater than 6 mm. Trauma to the anterior teeth is also more common in sport-loving boys than in other groups.

Such malocclusions are usually treated during the pubertal growth spurt— usually around 12–15 years for boys (11–13 for girls). The commonest form of treatment is with functional appliances. These position the mandible forwards, the stretched soft tissues pull the mandible back toward the retruded position and these forces are transmitted via the appliance to the maxilla and upper teeth.

One evening, the dentist and his nurse were just saying goodbye to the last patient, sorting out the surgery, and planning to leave when Robert came running into the waiting room. Robert was followed by his mate, Jaz, who was carrying a tooth. Robert was white and looked very shaken and was holding his hands over his mouth.

'I got hit', he mumbled to the dentist through his hands, 'with the bat, the cricket bat'. The dentist's nurse ushered Robert into the surgery and got him to sit on the dental chair. She retrieved the tooth from Jaz, who had been alert enough to spot the tooth in the grass, wrap it in his handkerchief and run with Robert to the surgery. She washed it gently and popped the tooth into a bowl of saline.

Immature incisors are more easily 'knocked out' than fully formed anterior teeth, partly because the root has not yet fully formed and partly because young bone is more flexible than adult bone. Thus a blow to the teeth more readily expands the socket, thereby avulsing the tooth. If there are no medical contra-indications, and the child is cooperative, immature teeth which have been avulsed should be replanted. The only exception to this is if there is a Class II malocclusion with a large overjet (as is the case with Robert). In such a case consideration should be given to using the space created, by the loss of the tooth, to reduce the overjet. Loss of one incisor rarely gives a good aesthetic result but replanted teeth may be more prone to resorption if moved orthodontically, so utilizing the space is worth consideration.

The dentist asked Jaz, who was aged 8, what had happened. Jaz said that there had been an argument amongst the boys about whether Robert, who had been keeping wicket, had stumped Zachary Brown out. Zac had got cross, explained Jaz, when Rob said he was out, then Zac swung the bat and hit Robert round the face.

The dentist then went to see Robert, who was in the surgery with the nurse. Although he was pale and obviously in pain, he did not seem overly upset.

Children's responses to single-event violent trauma vary considerably. Reactions may show immediately post-trauma or some days or even weeks after the event. Fearfulness of the event reoccurring or lack of trust in adults are two common responses. Additional reactions are dependent on age. Children aged 5 years or less will be fearful of being separated from the parent after a trauma, demonstrate crying, wailing, repeated activity (e.g. rocking), trembling and being overly clinging. Regressive behaviours are common. Children may return to earlier behaviours such as thumb sucking and enuresis. Parents need to be advised to show calmness and reassurance to the child as the parents' reactions can influence markedly children of this age. Children aged 6 to

11 years may exhibit marked withdrawal, variable attention, and negative behaviour. School refusal is common as well as irritability, increased fearfulness, aggressive outbursts, and bouts of anger. Sleep disturbance can also be a feature. Somatic symptoms, such as headaches or stomach aches with little or no organic confirmation, may be present. Features of mental health problems may be apparent such as depression, anxiety, or feelings of blame. In adolescents aged 12 to 17 years the common features displayed after a traumatic event are similar to those of adults. These include: depression, flashbacks, nightmares, numbing of emotional response, antisocial behaviour, poor sleep, and difficulties at school with academic work and relations with staff and peers. Avoiding school and the situation where the trauma took place are common aspects of trauma reactions.

Robert may show delayed reaction and will recover more quickly with support from his parents. The dentist should invite Robert to recount in his own words what had happened. Expressions of support by the dentist would be helpful. Let Robert know that it is normal to be upset following such an incident. Encourage the friend to provide his observations of the events leading up to the loss of Robert's tooth. Attempt to be non-judgemental while listening to Robert and also his friend. Advise the parent of the full circumstances of the events and recommend that the parent spend extra time, if at all possible, during the next 24 h to be with Robert. The gradual return to the normal routine in the family is to be welcomed and may be reassuring for the child. The parent might be advised to respect the preference of the child to keep the episode to themselves; however, the parent needs to inform the child that they, the parent(s), are always willing to discuss any difficulties their child experiences. There is every reason that Robert will recover quite quickly from the 'playground' incident. However, there is a need for the dentist to be able to identify those children that may require more intensive assistance and be able to refer on to specialized forms of psychotherapy.

'Okay Rob', the dentist asked, 'what happened?'

'Oh, I was wicket keeping and he went to take a huge shot. I was too close, and got hit.'

The dentist has been told differing versions of the events behind Robert's injury. The version put forward by Jaz, aged just 8 years, suggests that Robert was hit with a cricket bat deliberately by one Zachary Brown. On Robert's own account, it was an accident which happened because he got too close to the batsman. In the circumstances the dentist would be wise to record both versions in the notes. It is very unlikely that anything further would happen as a result of this accident or otherwise. Good note keeping is simply prudent.

The dentist ascertained from Robert that there had been little delay in coming to the surgery, although Robert said he had fallen to the floor and wasn't sure how long he had lain there. The dentist checked with Jaz, who said that Robert had got straight up.

The dentist is clearly hampered in ascertaining precisely what happened, in particular whether or not Robert was knocked out. Robert knows that he fell to the floor but does not remember how long he lay there. However, having sustained a heavy blow, it is not at all surprising that this poor lad is a bit vague on the details.

His little friend, Jaz, says Robert got up immediately. There is obviously some concern about Jaz's reliability as he is only 8 years old.

There can be no question that if the dentist is uncertain as to whether or not Robert was knocked out then a referral for medical attention is essential (see below). That is not an ethical or legal opinion. It is a matter of proper clinical judgement and a matter of common sense, which if not followed might bear some legal consequences, but such consequences would not be the reason for such referral.

In the absence of the mother this might require a referral to his GP's out of hours service if his GP is known, or to hospital by ambulance. However, when the mother eventually arrives it could be considered that the dentist's duty would be discharged by strongly advising the mother to call Robert's doctor or to take him to hospital, and possibly assisting her in making such arrangements.

The dentist tried to find out who else had been there but Rob seemed a bit vague about the answer to this question.

Robert has clearly received a severe blow to the face and possibly his head. In all cases where there is a head or face injury, the possibility of skull fracture or subdural haematoma formation must be considered. It is essential therefore to determine whether or not consciousness has been lost. If it has, then Robert should be referred to hospital for observation and possibly radiographic examination. The fact that Robert does not seem to remember the incident well is important. It would appear that he possibly did lose consciousness and that he has a slight degree of amnesia. The dentist should certainly have considered sending him to hospital. Some authorities advocate doing cranial nerve function tests, such as shining a torch into the eyes and checking pupil reaction. However, it remains clear that if the dentist suspects that head injury has been sustained, it is always best to have the child checked over by medically qualified staff. Other symptoms after a blow to the head, such as vomiting, headache, confusion, disorientation, or cerebrospinal leakage from the nose or ears are of course very significant. Patients exhibiting such symptoms should be immediately referred to hospital as emergencies.

In any case of trauma to the dentition, the dentist must ascertain the length of time which has elapsed between the injury being sustained and presentation to the dentist. In the case of avulsed teeth, the length of time out of the mouth is indirectly proportional to the chances of successful replantation. In the case of fractured teeth (see below) the probability of pulp death following an exposure is directly proportional to the length of time between injury and treatment.

One of the things the dentist should also do is to ensure that Robert does not have any facial fractures.

To check for zygomatic arch fracture:

- Look for depression of the malar (stand behind the seated patient and compare the shape of the right and left malars).
- Palpate bony landmarks for tenderness and deformity.
- Check mandibular function.
- Test for the presence of infraorbital anaesthesia.
- Test visual acuity using a piece of text.
- Test for diplopia by moving an object in the standard nine positions of gaze and asking about diplopia in each position.
- Pupil reactivity/light reflexes—using a pen torch/ophthalmoscope.

To check for mandibular fracture:

- Inspection.
- Palpate from condyle to condyle extra-orally.
- Palpate intra-orally.
- Look for sublingual haematoma, fracture movement, and mobile teeth.
- Check occlusion.
- Check mental nerve sensation.

Given that Robert seemed not to be too badly hurt, the dentist then suggested that he examine his teeth whilst the nurse tried to ring Robert's mother. The dentist knew that although Robert's father still lived in the village, he was divorced from Robert's mother.

'She's not in', said Rob. 'She's gone to the supermarket. She'll be about an hour and a half.'

'Well, who's looking after you?' asked the nurse.

'I hate going to the supermarket so mum always says that I can stay and play on the green 'til she gets back.'

The nurse then thought to ask:

'Where's your dad then?'

'Dunno', was the reply, 'but my gran's number is 0483.'

The dentist decided that he would go ahead and examine Robert's mouth anyway and Robert seemed happy about this.

Rob's lower lip was bruised and swollen with two small lacerations on the oral surface. He had a graze on his chin and his left cheek.

Robert's mother had left him to play while she went to the supermarket. Robert is only 9 years old. There appear to be no arrangements for any supervision for Robert. However, there is no law that states the minimum age that a child can be left alone. There is an offence of wilful neglect if parents leave a child unsupervised 'in a manner likely to cause unnecessary suffering or injury to health' (Children and Young Person's Act 1933). In Robert's case, it is unlikely that any offence has been committed or at least not one which would be success-fully prosecuted. However, leaving a group of young children playing cricket unsupervised, and with a very hard bat, is somewhat risky.

The dentist has been presented with an unaccompanied 9-year-old boy who needs urgent help and has come to him for it. Generally in life there is no moral requirement to be a 'good Samaritan'. It would be too onerous a burden on us all to spend our time doing good for others. Doing good is not an absolute moral obligation, in the same way as not harming others is. It usually does not require any positive action to fulfil the obligation not to do harm and therefore it is not particularly onerous to fulfil.

The situation here is, however, very different. First, there is a relationship between the dentist and Robert; he is a long-standing patient. Where a relationship exists there can be a moral duty to help others. The extent of that duty depends upon the relationship and the help required. Second, even in the absence of that relationship the dentist is professionally qualified to give the assistance Robert requires. There is no doubt that the dentist has a moral obligation to help Robert and such help will inevitably involve the provision of treatment.

What is the legal position? Robert is unaccompanied and therefore the issue of consent must be considered as the dentist must be sure that any treatment he provides is being carried out lawfully.

It is very likely that despite the divorce that Robert's father would still have 'parental responsibility' for Robert and be able to give consent to any dental treatment; however, he is not immediately contactable as Robert has no telephone number for him.

No attempt was made to contact Robert's grandmother, but in any event it is not at all certain that she would be in a position to give a valid consent to treatment, even if she had been contacted.

There are two provisions within the Children Act 1989 in respect of making decisions, which would include consent for dental treatment, for children by persons who do not have 'parental responsibility'.

First, under section 2 (9): a person who has parental responsibility for a child may not surrender or transfer any part of that responsibility to another but may arrange for some or all of it to be met by one or more persons acting on his behalf. Such a situation would arise if, say, the mother had sent Robert to the dentist along with grandmother. That is not the case here.

Second, under section 3 (5) a person who (a) does not have parental responsibility for a particular child but (b) has care of the child may do what is reasonable in all the circumstances of the case for the purpose of safeguarding or promoting the child's welfare. Again that is not the case here, as the grandmother had not been left in charge of Robert.

What about Robert himself. Can he give a valid consent? He is only 9 years old. Children below the age of 16 years can consent to their own dental treatment provided that they have reached a sufficient understanding and intelligence to be capable of making up their own mind on the matter. (Gillick v West Norfolk and Wisbech Area Health Authority [1985] 3 All ER 402)—hence the term 'Gillick competent child'.

Is Robert 'Gilllick competent'? He has realized straightaway that he needs help and has recognized, and gone to, the very person who can best assist him. He has even had, or perhaps his little friend has had, the presence of mind to bring the avulsed tooth with him. Such would indicate a good basis for 'Gillick competence'. It seems that the dentist has explained very clearly to Robert what needs to done and, hopefully, why. Such would satisfy the very basic requirements of the nature and purpose of the treatment. There is an initial reluctance regarding the injection—that is overcome by answers to Robert's questions about it and some encouragement from his little friend. Treatment seems to have then proceeded without any problems or complaint. It seems that Robert was entirely compliant. Robert therefore would seem to have given a lawfully valid consent to the reimplantation of the UR1 and dressing of UL1 and splinting of UR2 and UR1.

However, if Robert were not 'Gillick competent', would the dentist's moral and professional duty to help Robert be supported by law? The answer is 'Yes'. The dentist would be permitted to provide treatment in these circumstances under the 'doctrine of necessity'. The doctrine arises from the inability to communicate with a person who is able to consent and that there is insufficient time to wait until such communication can take place. It does not arise necessarily because there is an emergency situation, although it often does, and it does not require the necessary treatment to be life-saving. In this clinical situation, the sooner the tooth is reimplanted the better its prognosis. The prospects of success diminish each minute the tooth is out of the socket. If the dentist is not happy to proceed with Robert's consent and he waits for the mother then the chances of successful reimplantation diminish with each minute that passes. Thus, the dentist is already acting in Robert's best interests by proceeding with treatment as soon as possible.

Of course, the dentist must only provide that treatment which is essential to protect Robert's immediate welfare. The treatment must be treatment which is in Robert's best interests. Whether or not a treatment is in a patient's best interest is determined by the 'accepted practice test' or the 'Bolam test'.

In a landmark case for the provision of treatment to incompetent adult patients unable to consent for themselves it was said that not only would it be lawful to carry out treatment in the absence of consent but that there would be a legal duty to do so (F v West Berkshire Health Authority [1989] 2 All ER 545).

When a person sustains a blow to the mouth area, particularly if it is sustained by a fall in which the face comes into contact with the ground, it is common for the lips to be lacerated. This is also common in cases where a tooth has been broken. It is essential, if teeth are fractured, to try to account for the tooth fragments. Occasionally, the fragment may be within the lip. Therefore, if there is a fractured tooth and lacerations to the lip, a soft tissue profile radiograph should be taken. Tooth fragments in the soft tissue will show as non-anatomical radiodensities. If teeth or tooth fragments are missing and the patient thinks they may have swallowed the tooth, a chest X-ray is advisable to ensure that the tooth has not been inhaled. Teeth which are inhaled are usually located in the left lung as the left main bronchus is more vertical than the right. Inhaled teeth and tooth fragments can potentially lead to lung abscess and therefore must be dealt with promptly.

Should a tooth fragment be detected in the lip, a second radiograph may be needed to determine its precise location. If the fragment lies close to the surface, simply stretching and everting the lip at the fragment site should make it appear from the laceration. Otherwise, surgical removal under local anaesthesia plus antibiotics may be required.

Severe lacerations to the lips, particularly at the junction of the vermilion border with the skin, should be repaired with utmost care, preferably by a plastic surgeon, as scarring and poor aesthetic results are problematic in this area.

Examining a child who has been involved in an accident, and who has sustained physical damage, is difficult. The child is likely to be upset and the parents, if present, will be shocked and anxious. The situation requires a calm, soothing, but efficient attitude on behalf of the dentist.

It is important to begin the examination by asking the patient when, where, and how the accident happened. The length of time between injury and presentation, as explained above, can affect the choice of treatment. If the wound is contaminated with soil, a tetanus injection may be indicated and the whereabouts of the event is obviously of crucial importance if a tooth has been completely avulsed and lost. All teeth and tooth fragments should be accounted for. As mentioned earlier, if there is any doubt about possible inhalation, a chest X-ray should be arranged. A precise description of the accident will give the dentist an idea of how severe an impact the child has sustained and therefore will help in the assessment of the severity of any other injuries.

Clear and detailed contemporaneous notes should be kept, documenting all the above facts. This will be invaluable to the dentist should a court case arise from the injuries.

The dentist should also take a medical history and enquire specifically about symptoms related to the accident, such as consciousness, amnesia, vomiting, and headache.

If examination reveals that the patient is disorientated or less alert than usual they should be referred to hospital. The facial area should be inspected for injuries and the facial bones palpated for signs of fracture or displacement. In particular, limitation of jaw movement should be investigated.

Intraorally all soft tissues, the periodontium, and the occlusion should be checked. The extent of tooth fractures (whether involving enamel, dentine, or pulp), tooth displacement, and evidence of alveolar fracture should be noted.

Once the initial examination has been completed, periapical radiographs (preferably two at different angles) should be taken of any traumatized teeth, plus a soft tissue view of the lip if there are lacerations and tooth fragments are unaccounted for. If facial fractures are suspected, appropriate films should be taken.

Radiographs should be carefully examined for 'non-obvious' injuries, such as root and alveolar fractures.

The upper right central incisor was missing—presumably the tooth which Jaz had been carrying which was now residing in the bowl of saline. The upper right lateral incisor was extremely mobile and had been displaced palatally. Its position meant that Robert could not close his back teeth together. The upper left central incisor was fractured. The fracture ran from the mesial edge, almost at the gingival level, to the disto-incisal corner through enamel denture and pulp. The pulpal exposure was approximately 1 mm in diameter. The upper left lateral incisor had a enamel fracture on the incisal edge.

The dentist told Robert that he could put the tooth back in place, but that he would need to have an injection. Robert was not particularly happy about this, but, having asked questions about whether it would hurt, agreed to try.

In a study in the northwest of England with 313 children aged 8–15 years it was found that 35% stated that they were 'very afraid' of the local anaesthetic injection. This compares with 19% and 18% of the children rating tooth extraction or inhalation sedation in the same way. Only 8% were very afraid of having a filling. Hence the injection was found to be the most anxiety-provoking procedure. It is also clear that children who participate in surveys to ascertain their anxiety to various dental procedures are most anxious at the younger end of the age range. Many of the surveys of children who rely on self-report (and not the mothers' ratings) start at 8 years of age, Robert, who is 9 years at the time of this incident, is likely to be afraid of an injection. He has not had previous dental treatment. The receipt of an injection would therefore be a new experience in addition to the shock of having a tooth knocked out by a cricket bat. The dentist would need to explain that the procedure of having an injection could be made with little discomfort by the use of topical anaesthetic gel. Paradoxically, it has been shown that 9- to 12-year-old children who have not had any dental treatment experience will tend to be more dentally anxious.

Jaz helped to encourage Robert's decision by saying how he'd had injections at the dentist and that it hadn't hurt. The dentist therefore anaesthetized the UR1 socket, replanted the tooth and aligned the UR2. He also placed calcium hydroxide on the pulpal exposure and the dentine on UL1 and placed a composite bandage on the tooth.

In cases of trauma to immature incisor teeth, the primary objective of treatment is to promote root formation by, if at all possible, maintaining the vitality of the pulp, particularly the radicular pulp. If this fails, then the treatment objective is still to try to achieve root end closure. Thus, unless the pulp is clearly infected and damaged, indirect pulp capping is worth trying. After such treatment, the dentist will need to take radiographs at regular intervals to ensure that the root is forming.

If a pulp exposure is large (>2 mm) or if the pulpal tissue has been in contact with the mouth for long enough to ensure infection (4–5 h) then removal of the coronal pulp is advisable (pulpotomy). This requires a local anaesthetic (this should provide immediate relief to the patient as the pulp will be extremely sensitive). The dentine surrounding the exposure and the coronal pulp are then removed. This is best done with a conventional handpiece as the air rotor's water may contaminate the pulp.

Once bleeding has stopped, calcium hydroxide is placed on the pulpal exposure, the dentine etched with a normal etching solution or gel, washed, dried, and composite applied either freehand or using an acetate crown form to build a tooth-shaped composite tip.

If the tooth root does not form, or the radicular pulp becomes non-vital, or periapical pathology is visible on radiographs, the necrotic radicular pulp will have to be removed and non-setting calcium hydroxide paste spun into the root canal. This should be replaced every 3 months. After 9–18 months, an 'apex' should have formed at the distal end of the tooth (see later).

The replanted UR1 and mobile UR2 were splinted to UL1 and UL2. More stable splinting was not possible as neither the canines nor the premolar teeth had yet erupted.

The nurse sat with Jaz who, just as the dentist was finishing the work, pointed and said: 'There's Rob's mum.'

The nurse rushed out on to the green and said: 'I'm afraid Robert has had a little accident'.

Robert's mother blanched and she wobbled on her feet.

'Oh, he's okay, he's okay, it's just his teeth.'

'His teeth', his mum cried. 'His lovely new teeth.'

The nurse ushered Robert's mother towards the dental practice. Just as they came through the main door, Robert and the dentist emerged from the surgery.

Robert's mother hugged Robert and the dentist explained what he had done and what Robert had said had happened. The dentist then took Robert's mother to one side and explained that Jaz's story had been a little different from Robert's. The dentist suggested that she might wish to make further enquiries from Robert's friends.

Robert and his mother then went home, with an appointment to return in a week's time. As it was now quite late in the evening, the dentist thought he would write up Robert's notes the following day.

The essence of good note keeping is that the notes should be full and con-temporaneous. This is a professional obligation (General Dental Council 'Main-taining standards'). It would be better that the dentist wrote the notes that evening when the events were still fresh in his memory. There is a danger that by leaving it until the following day those events of the previous evening will not be recorded so accurately.

There are three main types of record used commonly in clinical practice. They are: cognitive record, written record, and computer record. Cognitive record, or in other words committing the detail to memory, has the advantages of being quick and requiring little effort. Certain facts can be held in memory that appear significant at the time, and information that is considered not important can be released from memory. It also has the advantage of being able to link to other simi-lar events or patients to form patterns that confirm a particular view about a den-tal health problem and its causation or treatment approach. In this way the information collected is truly relational, in that the case material is very often asso-ciated with similar circumstances or patients seen at other times. Hence the social impressions of the interaction between the patient and dentist may survive but the matters of fact are poorly retained to memory. It may appear, at first, cost-effective as little time is required for this process of record 'keeping' and can be managed at the same time as other routine activities are being conducted. Unfortunately there are many disadvantages including the obvious one of proneness to memory faults. In the short term the clinician can retain a comparatively large amount of infor-mation. However, with continual contact with new or repeat patients the prob-ability of retention reduces. The information that is retained is subject to bias and can become disorganized, or error prone, as details of other patients become mixed with the case under attention or investigation. At worst the holder of the cognitive record can become ill or even die, and what details are held are lost.

The written record performs two functions: first to ensure continuity of care and secondly to act in medico-legal cases to support the clinical judgements and practice of the clinician. It has the advantage of the record surviving if stored properly, is cheap to produce on paper, and can be standardized in the format of collating information to assist with speedy retrieval. There is also a familiarity which aids access. Storage is an issue requiring care to protect the confidentiality of the patient and a systematic approach to identifying the author by signature and date is required.

A computer record can improve the legibility of the records and help to standardize entry of information and retrieval. Audit and research can be facilitated by the use of computer records but issues of security and confidentiality must be given due consideration. Costs of space, equipment, training, maintenance, depreciation, support, storage, and backup are all important.

Some essential points, apart from information about medical and dental history, for written record keeping include:

- Write detailed and contemporaneous notes clearly and legibly.
- The patient's name and date must appear on each card or sheet of record.
- All telephone conversations with the patient and family members should be recorded.
- Separate factual data from opinions.
- Alterations must be declared by signature.
- Take care when including sensitive information about patients, with preference for facts or observations.
- Be careful not to use derogatory terms about patients.
- Be sure to include: when consent was obtained and the capacity of the patient to give consent, and also only include information that you could state under oath in court of law.

Later that evening, the dentist became increasingly concerned that he had witnessed the results of a quite vicious assault. He became so worried about this that eventually he telephoned the police and reported what had happened.

The following week, Robert and his mother attended for Robert's appointment. Robert's mum was angry. Firstly, the police had been to her house as a result of the dentist's phone call. She was most distressed that the police had become involved in an incident in which, according to her was 'boys being boys'. Another reason she was annoyed was because, for the last two nights, Robert had been kept awake by intense pain from both of the central incisor teeth.

'I wish you'd never put that tooth back in. It's causing trouble and I know it's going to end up being more trouble than it's worth.'

The dentist tried to explain the reasons he replanted Robert's tooth, to which the mother replied that: 'you should never have done it without my say so'.

The issue of whether the dentist acted correctly by treating Robert in his mother's absence has been dealt with earlier. It is particularly relevant here to consider what complaints might be made against the dentist if he had *not* reimplanted the tooth and the mother had found out that this was the best treatment option in the circumstances.

The dentist recognized that the teeth were pulpitic, probably irreversibly so. He explained to Robert and his mother that he would need to remove the pulps from the teeth and put something in the teeth to help the root to form.

Pain which is stimulated by changes in temperature implies that the pulp of the tooth is inflamed and hyperaemic. If pain occurs spontaneously, this can indicate that eventually the inflammation will become so intense that the pulpal blood supply will be compromised and the pulp will become necrotic. This point, when the pulp is inflamed and is going to die but is still vital and causing pain, is sometimes known as 'irreversible pulpitis'. However, it is unwise to suppose that it is possible to distinguish the histological differences between 'reversible' and 'irreversible' pulpitis simply by taking a pain history.

In Robert's case, the teeth had become progressively worse since the initial treatment. Leaving him in such pain was not an option, so the dentist had no choice other than to remove the pulps of the teeth and attempt apexification (see above). This involves placing calcium hydroxide in the root canal in an attempt to stimulate the apical tissue into creating a hard tissue apex to the tooth, despite root formation being incomplete. If root end closure can be achieved, root canal treatment will be possible.

The epithelial root sheath of Hertwig is the entity which enables the peri-apical tissues of non-vital teeth to continue root formation. This tissue appears to be able sometimes to fulfil its function even in the absence of a healthy pulp. Stimulation of the epithelial cells can result in dentine being laid down across the open apex of the tooth. Alternatively, cementocytes may be able to grow from undamaged root and thereby calcific repair of the apex with cementum is achieved. Apical closure is therefore either the result of continued root development, or calcific scarring. The latter is thought to be promoted by the presence of calcium hydroxide. Even incomplete root end closure makes root filling the tooth much easier. The 'blunderbuss' shape of an immature root makes root filling very difficult unless some apexification is carried out.

The dentist proceeded to extirpate the central incisors under local anaesthetic, noticing as he did so that although UR2 had firmed up well, UR1 did not appear to be any more stable than when he had just replanted it.

Despite weekly visits, repeated splinting and 3-monthly applications of CaOH to the root canal, UR1 failed to become firm. After 9 months, UR1 was extracted and a single tooth denture provided for Robert.

Design of dentures

In designing dentures the following steps may be followed:
- Saddle—outline the teeth to be replaced.
- Connector—decide on the type and design of connector.
- Support—elements in the denture, such as rest seats, that resist vertical forces directed to the mucosa.
- Retention—provide adequate retention: directly through the use of clasps, mucosal coverage and muscular forces and indirectly to provide further resistance to movement.

In this situation we are replacing a single central incisor in a 10-year-old with an increased overjet. The first denture will probably be an immediate replacement. Normally this will be an acrylic plate, possibly with simple stainless steel clasps such as Adams' clasps on the first molars. Socketing of the denture should not be provided but a flange will aid retention and disguise early alveolar bone loss. Gingival relief of 4 mm should be provided around the other teeth. On providing immediate dentures, patients should be advised that such prostheses are temporary and will normally require relining or replacement within the first year. In this case, Robert will continue to grow for several more years and will require several dentures, probably of similar design.

At this point, the calcific barrier at the apex of UL1 was considered well developed. The tooth was root filled.

Once apexification has been achieved, the tooth will need to be root filled. The materials for doing this are normal sealant and gutta percha. However, the canal of an immature tooth will be wider than the thickest master point. Thus, when root treating such teeth a lateral condensation technique is important. The technique involves firstly choosing a master gutta percha point which best fits the canal. This point should be sealed into the canal, then the steel prong of a lateral spreader is pushed in between the point and the canal wall. The point is then adapted (squashed) firmly against part of the canal wall. Removal of the spreader leaves a space into which an accessory gutta percha point can be introduced, it having been coated, before insertion, with sealer. This process should be repeated until it is not possible to place any further gutta percha points. Ten or twelve points may be needed. Care should be taken to avoid excessive lateral pressure as the root walls of the immature incisor may be thin and fragile.

Robert and his mother then voiced increasing concern about Robert's 'goofy' appearance. Robert said that he is teased at school and called names because of his protruding front teeth.

Robert's malocclusion could be treated, despite the denture, with functional appliances, although he is a little young at 10 to commence this treatment. It is more usual to await eruption of the premolar teeth before commencing treatment.

The alternative which an orthodontist might suggest is that the denture is left out (the patient's reaction to this suggestion must be gauged, as clearly aesthetic appearance will be severely compromised by such a course of action). Having no denture will allow mesial drift of the lateral incisor. If space closure is the preferred option, this drift could be encouraged with appliances. With an overjet as large as Robert's, the orthodontist might also suggest extraction of the first premolar on the side opposite to the lost UR1, in order to try to get symmetrical reduction of the overjet. The ultimate aim of such treatment would be to crown, or do a composite build-up on, the centrally placed UR2, in order to try to make it appear like the avulsed UR1 and similarly to alter the shape of UR3 to more closely mimic the appearance of an incisor tooth.

The size and morphology of the UR2 would be of great importance when deciding whether allowing space closure, as described above, would be a sensible option. Likewise, the patient's cooperation with functional appliances may prove to be the deciding factor when deciding whether to allow space closure or not.

Robert also says that the denture 'looks horrible' and 'made it impossible' for him to play the flute which he had started learning. The dentist therefore referred Robert to an orthodontist.

Fortunately, Robert did not have crowding in either arch and the orthodontist wrote back to the dentist to say that he would treat Robert with a
functional appliance.

Had Robert's mouth been crowded, the second option (allowing the space to
close, then altering the appearance of UR2, UR3) would be preferred. If spacing were present in the maxilla, functional appliance therapy would be preferred. However, the patient's ability to wear such an appliance, along with a
denture, whilst maintaining his/her oral hygiene (rarely excellent in 10-year-
old boys) would be a crucial element in the decision-making process.

The orthodontist thought Robert would cope with the functional appliance and the denture at the same time. However, he also expressed concern that the short root on UL1 may make it more than usually liable to
resorption.

Robert continued to have good oral health other than his malocclusion and
the problems with the denture. When he was 16, the dentist suggested that the
denture could be replaced with a resin-retained bridge.

There are a number of different fitting surface treatments for resin-retained
bridges but the common types are sand-blasting and acid or electrolytic etching (the latter type is called a Maryland bridge). The Rochette bridge relies on
mechanical retention from holes in the framework and, although no longer
popular, still has a limited role as an interim restoration, perhaps during or
prior to implant work. The success rate of resin-retained bridges can be high
but careful attention must be paid to design, surface treatment, and adhesion.
The design most likely to succeed is a single cantilever. Before providing a resin-
retained bridge the following factors should be taken into account: spacing,
occlusion, restoration of adjacent teeth, bone support, numbers of other teeth
present, and the condition of the mouth.

An implant is being planned for Robert, so a Rochette type bridge may
be chosen as an intermediate restoration that may subsequently be removed
without too much difficulty.

This would then be followed, once Robert's jaw has stopped growing, by a
single tooth implant.

There are only some patients and circumstances in which an implant is
an appropriate treatment. Implants are *not* a suitable treatment modality if
the patient is severely medically compromised or too young (i.e. still growing).
Furthermore, the following factors would also contra-indicate placement of an
implant:
- insufficient space (at least 5 mm are required mesio-distally)
- insufficient bone
- high exposure to tobacco smoke
- bruxism
- poor patient compliance.

An implant is considered to be successful if the following clinical criteria are achieved:
- An individual, unattached implant is immobile when tested clinically.
- Radiographic examination does not reveal any peri-implant radio-lucency.
- After the first year in function, radiographic bone loss is less than 0.2 mm per annum.
- The individual implant performance is characterized by an absence of signs and symptoms such as pain, infections, neuropathies, paraesthesia, or violation of the inferior dental canal.
- As a minimum, if an implant fulfils the above criteria in 85% of cases at the end of 5 years and 80% of cases at the end of 10 years it would be deemed to be a successful implant/operator system.

The following procedure should be followed if an implant is being considered:
- Examination of appearance and function.
- Evaluation of the edentulous area. This can be done simply by visual assessment and palpation. In addition, the bone contour can be mapped out on a sectioned stone cast using measurements taken of the soft tissues with callipers or a graduated probe.

  Radiographs are also required to assess bone width, contour, and quality.
- Study casts and diagnostic wax-ups are used to determine the number and position of teeth to be replaced and the occlusal relationship. They can then be used for radiographic and surgical stents and for the construction of temporary restorations.

This is followed by surgical placement of the implant, which then undergoes osseointegration. Once this has occurred, the implant prosthesis can be placed.

Thus, at aged 21 an implant was placed to replace UR1.

For years, Robert's implant was fine, then, suddenly, aged 27, he noticed that the tooth had become mobile.

Mobility in implants

Implants are more likely to become mobile if the following apply:
- Poor bone quality with sparse trabeculation. Failure rates may be higher for implants placed in bone with thin cortex, low trabecular density, and poor medullary strength.
- Loading. Occlusal interferences and overloading may contribute to implant failure.
- Smoking. Failure rates are generally higher with increased tobacco exposure. The failure rates are higher in the maxilla than in the mandible.
- Peri-implant infections. These are less common in patients with good oral hygiene.

Eventually, the decision was made that the implant would have to be removed. The treatment options at this stage were:
- re-implant
- ceramic bridge
- adhesive bridges
- denture.

Robert and the dentist discussed the options. Robert asked his dentist for more information on the relative longevity of each of the options.

Comparison of the longevity of bridges and implants shows the following:
- For conventional bridges, a meta-analysis of fixed partial denture (bridge) prostheses and abutments showed that one-third of all bridges require replacement by 15 years (Scurria *et al.* 1998).
- For resin-retained bridges: the median survival time for such bridges is over 7 years.
- Implants are said to have approximately 90% survival at 10 years, whilst dentures normally have a lifespan of an average of 5 years, depending on bone resorption rates.

Eventually, after much discussion, Robert decided that he preferred a bridge to the alternative treatments.

One of the problems in providing a bridge in this case is the substantial bone loss in the area of the edentulous ridge where the implant failed and was subsequently removed. It is difficult to disguise the bone loss using a bridge. If the patient has a low lip line, the long pontic will not be seen but this can be a problem for patients with high lip lines. In such cases, attempts can be made to disguise the length of the pontic by using pink porcelain at the neck or by providing a removable flange. Bone grafting prior to bridgework provision could also be considered. Dentures have the advantage of being able to replace soft and hard tissue as well as teeth.

For a missing UR1, with UL1 root filled and with a short root, the bridge treatment options for Robert are as follows:
- Resin retained cantilever from UL1: The problem with this option is, what happens if root canal treatment in UL1 fails? In this case this eventuality would appear to be highly unlikely as the tooth has been root filled for several years without any complications. However, the dentist should carefully consider whether or not the short-rooted UL1 will be able to take the load.
- Resin retained cantilever from UR2: The problem with this bridge design is that it would need a large surface area of enamel for bonding and favourable occlusion. Lateral incisors are often small teeth and it therefore may not be of adequate size.
- Conventional cantilever from UL1: Again, the suitability of this design depends on how likely the root canal treatment on the UL1 is to remain

problem free (but see the first option). If occlusion is unfavourable, excess loading could possibly explain why the implant failed.

- Conventional fixed–fixed from UR2 and UL1: This design would involve preparation of the UR2, which is a sound tooth. However, if the above options were not possible for the reasons described, this might be a suitable option.
- Fixed–moveable from UR2 and UL1 with moveable joint between UL1 and UR1: This might be a suitable design but such joints can be bulky and technically this is a more difficult treatment to accomplish.
- Combination—conventional retainer on UL1 with resin-retained wing on UR2: The problem here would be that you would need to design for failure of the resin-retained wing, therefore you would need a moveable joint between UR1 and UL1.
- Combination—conventional retainer on UR2 with resin-retained wing on UL1: The problem again is that you have to design for failure of the resin-retained wing and therefore need a moveable joint between UR2 and UR1. This design would again involve preparation of the unrestored UR2.

Three weeks later, the dentist started Robert's treatment.

A bridge requires that dentist carefully choose the appropriate shade. Facebow and occlusal records as well as study casts will be required.

Tooth preparation under local anaesthesia will be followed by an accurate impression being taken using a silicone-based impressive material. A temporary bridge is made for the patient to wear until the definitive prosthesis has been made.

Ten years later, Robert's bridge is intact. He is a regular dental attender and now brings his family along for dental check-ups. Robert is assiduous in the care of his children's teeth, presumably because of the problems his dental injury caused him.

The dentist is careful to offer appropriate advice. This includes encouragement of brushing the children's teeth with a fluoride toothpaste.

The dentist has also warned Robert about the possibility of his children requiring orthodontic treatment as they get older, as facial growth to some extent follows a familial pattern. Finally, the dentist advises that Robert's children should wear mouthguards when playing contact sports.

If Robert chooses to have mouth guards made by the dentist for his children he will have to pay privately for them. It would be possible for him to buy mouth guards ready made from a good sports shop or he could purchase the 'boil in the bag' type of mouthguard kit, which moulds itself to the patient's teeth. These tend to be more retentive and better fitting than the 'off the rack' mouth guards but are still not as effective, comfortable, or retentive as the mouth guards made by dentists.

Robert's two children grow up with intact dentitions but both require orthodontic treatment with functional and fixed appliances when they reach their early teenage years.

Facial growth patterns and, in particular, skeletal patterns are familial. Thus, a parent with a jaw-to-jaw discrepancy is likely to see the same facial features in his/her children. Class II malocclusions can be successfully treated by growth modification using functional appliances and removable appliances can be used to correct the protrusion of maxillary teeth caused by habits. However, if bodily tooth movement is required then fixed appliances will be needed. Thus, the child will need to be referred to an orthodontist.

BIBLIOGRAPHY

Andreasen J. *Essentials of Traumatic Injuries to the Teeth*, 2nd edn. Munksgaard: Copenhagen, 2000.

el-Mowafy O, Rubo MH. Resin-bonded fixed dentures—a literature review with presentation of a novel approach. *International Journal of Prosthodontics* 2000; **13**(6): 460–467.

F v West Berkshire Health Authority [1989] 2 All ER 545

General Dental Council. *Maintaining Standards.* www.gdc-uk.org/pdfs/ms_full_nov2001.pdf

Gillick v West Norfolk and Wisbech Area Health Authority [1095] 3 All ER 402.

McCloskey LA, Walker M. Posttraumatic stress in children exposed to family violence and single-event trauma. *Journal of the American Academy of Child and Adolescent Psychiatry* 2000; **39**(1): 108–115.

Murray P, Liddell A, Donohue J. A longitudinal study of the contribution of dental experience to dental anxiety in children between 9 and 12 years of age. *Journal of Behavioral Medicine* 1989; **12**(3): 309–320.

Palmer RM. *A Clinical Guide to Implants in Dentistry.* BDJ Books: London, 2000.

Scurria MS, Bader JD, Shugars DA. Meta-analysis of fixed partial denture survival: prostheses and abutments. *Journal of Prosthetic Dentistry* 1998; **79**(4): 459–464.

Tips on ... clinical record keeping. *British Medical Journal* 2002; **325**: S23.

Wong G, Humphris GM, Lee GTR. Preliminary validation and reliability of the Modified Child Dental Anxiety Scale. *Psychological Reports* 1998; **83**: 1179–1186.

6 Jess: the disappearing teeth

Jess is 5 years old. Her mother is a head teacher at a private girls' school and her father is a financial director for an international banking corporation. At 43 and 45, Jess's parents are at least 10 years older than the parents of the other children who go the same nursery school. Jess's mother is very health- and appearance-conscious. She is also very concerned about academic performance and tidiness.

Is Jess at high or low risk for dental disease?
How do we know which children get most disease?

Jess has been taken to the local dentist's surgery for check-ups since she was 6 months old. She has always been a timid yet precocious child and has always cooperated beautifully when she has been examined.

Jess's oral hygiene is exemplary. Her mother brushes her teeth for her twice every day.

Having never had any problems, the dentist was surprised when Jess's mother rang for an emergency appointment. When asked what the problem was, she replied that Jess's tooth was changing colour.

When examined, ULA was clearly darker than the other teeth.

What questions should the dentist ask about this tooth?

On questioning Jess's mother, there was no obvious cause for the tooth's discoloration. There was also no sinus, nor did a periapical radiograph show any radiolucency, other than that associated with the crypt of the developing UL1.

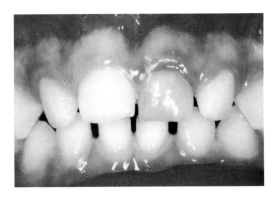

Discoloured URA

How should teeth with this appearance be treated?

In Jess's case, the dentist felt that the ULA was non-vital due to previous but unknown trauma and that it would therefore be better if it were removed so that the successor tooth would not be affected by any infection which might develop.

Does trauma to deciduous teeth affect the underlying permanent tooth?

The dentist informed Jess's mother that the tooth was dead and needed to be removed.

Is the patient/parent able to make an informed choice about the proposed treatment?

Jess's mother agreed to the extraction and the dentist prepared to remove the tooth under local anaesthesia. At the point of extraction, Jess became very very distressed, almost hysterical. However, Jess's mother insisted that the dentist continue and helped to hold Jess still. The dentist managed to extract the tooth but Jess was inconsolable.

Is restraint of small children for extractions acceptable and/or legal?
Should symptomless discoloured deciduous teeth always be extracted?

After the extraction, the UL1 erupted a little earlier than normal but appeared normal, apart from some white flecks. The contralateral tooth UR1 was not similarly affected.

What causes flecks in enamel?

At the age of 8, Jess attended for her 6-monthly check-up as usual. (Her mother had continued to bring her after the extraction, and after three or four visits in which she was cajoled into an examination, Jess once again became cooperative.) Jess complained at this visit of having 'funny teeth'.

Why might Jess believe her teeth to be abnormal?

When the dentist enquired further, Jess said that her teeth were 'all yellowy' and that they were 'goofy'. On examination, Jess's teeth and occlusion were normal. The dentist told Jess's mother that there was no cause for concern with Jess's teeth and that she did not need treatment.

Who should the dentist discuss his treatment plan with?

Jess's visits continued to be regular, and her oral hygiene perfect.

When Jess was about 12 years old, the dentist noticed that there was some gingival recession of the canine teeth.

Why does recession particularly occur on canine teeth?

When questioned, Jess explained that she did brush these teeth particularly carefully because, she said, they were very yellow. The dentist also noticed that the URE and ULE were showing no signs of exfoliation.

The dentist therefore took a periapical radiograph of each and discovered that UR5 and UL5 were missing.

Why are these premolars missing?
What can be done about the missing UR5, UL5?

The dentist advised Jess that she would have to look after her baby molar teeth very carefully, so that they would last. The dentist also made a brief note that Jess appeared to be rather under weight.

At the age of 14, Jess attended, looking extremely thin. She said that when she ate something cold, or even if very cold air got near to her teeth, they were painful. She also said that: her teeth were 'shrinking'. Her mother then said that she knew why Jess's teeth were getting shorter. She said she has read in the newspapers about soft drinks causing erosion. She asked the dentist to tell Jess to stop 'drinking all that rubbish'.

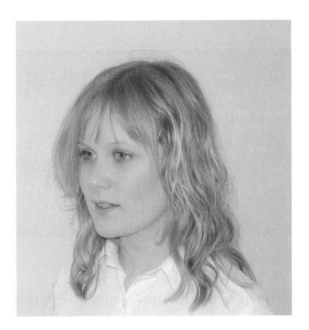

Jess

What disorder might be affecting Jess?
What can the dentist infer from the mother's behaviour?

Having listened to this rather strange history from Jess, the dentist tried to work out what was going on. On examination, he found that the incisal edges of Jess's teeth were thin and there was wear of the upper palatal surfaces. Also he could see wear facets on the cusps of the lower posterior teeth. The URE and ULE were completely smooth and at gingival level.

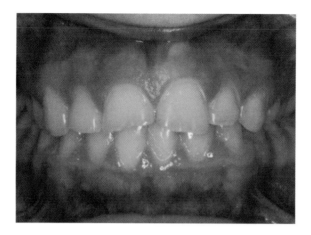

Erosion of upper incisors

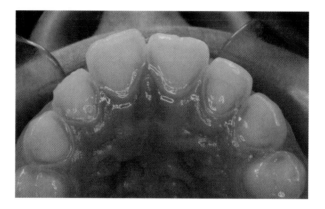

Palatal view of eroded incisors

What can we learn from the pattern of tooth surface loss?

The dentist decided that Jess's diet did indeed have something to do with her worn teeth, but decided that the best option, in the first instance, was to recommend that Jess use a desensitizing toothpaste and come back in a month.

How should dentine hypersensitivity be managed?

Jess's mother seemed unimpressed with this course of action but agreed to it, muttering about the 'rubbish Jess drank' as she left the surgery.

Why does Jess's mother think Jess drinks 'rubbish'?

After a month, Jess returned, but said that her teeth were 'still shrinking' and that there had not been any improvement in the sensitivity. On examination, the teeth looked much the same as on the previous occasion but the dentist could not be sure. At this point, the dentist considered what options were available for Jess.

What are the treatment options?

A treatment plan was drawn up in discussion with Jess (but not her mother who the dentist excluded from the discussion). When it was explained that food could affect her teeth, Jess agreed to see a dietician about her eating habits.

Jess's mother was very against Jess seeing anyone else about what she ate.

When she was 18, Jess went to the surgery to tell the dentist that she hated the appearance of the URE and ULE. These were worn down and discoloured, and Jess felt they were visible when she smiled. The dentist thought Jess looked well, although still slightly under weight.

What can be done about the retained teeth?

The URE and ULE were extracted and the spaces closed orthodontically. Jess then went to university. She had achieved extremely high grades at 'A' level and was going to study medicine. The dentist wondered whether he should alert the university authorities to Jess's eating disorder.

Should a dentist inform others about his patients' health problems?

Aged 24, Jess returned to the surgery saying that she was getting married in 3 months' time and that she definitely wanted her teeth made whiter and longer. On questioning she stated that she had not been able to complete her medical degree, after having had a year off after studying medicine for 2 years. She had decided that she may have chosen to do the medical degree for the wrong reasons, related more to the wishes of her parents rather than following her real interests.

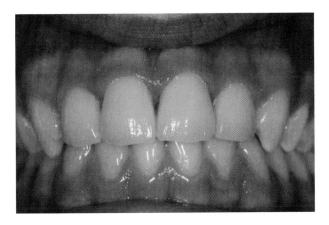

Upper incisors restored with resin bonded crowns

Can the dentist help Jess to achieve the appearance she desires?
Should the dentist be concerned about Jess's continued interest in improving the appearance of her teeth?

JESS: THE DISAPPEARING TEETH

Jess is 5 years old. Her mother is a head teacher at a private girls' school and her father is a financial director for an international banking corporation. At 43 and 45, Jess's parents are at least 10 years older than the parents of the other children who go the same nursery school. Jess's mother is very health- and appearance-conscious. She is also very concerned about academic performance and tidiness.

Dental caries experience is closely related to socioeconomic status. Children from deprived backgrounds have higher levels of decay, in both the primary and secondary dentitions, than their more affluent peers. This is known partly because of the decennial survey of both adults and children's teeth which have been carried out in the UK since 1968 (see Bibliography) and because of the child dental health surveys which are coordinated by the British Association for the Study of Community Dentistry (BASCD). This rolling programme of epidemiological studies examines 12, 5, 14 and 5-year-old children in successive years. Thus, we have a clear picture of the patterns of decay in children, particularly in 5-year-olds.

Jess has been taken to the local dentist's surgery for check-ups since she was 6 months old. She has always been a timid yet precocious child and has always cooperated beautifully when she has been examined.

Jess's oral hygiene is exemplary. Her mother brushes her teeth for her twice every day.

Having never had any problems, the dentist was surprised when Jess's mother rang for an emergency appointment. When asked what the problem was, she replied that Jess's tooth was changing colour.

When examined, ULA was clearly darker than the other teeth.

If a child presents with an apparently traumatic injury (and if an A is non-vital and non-carious trauma is very high on the list of possible causes) the dentist must take a clear history about how the injury occurred.

Often in very small children the tooth will have been knocked during the rough and tumble of the toddler years and very often the incident is overlooked as a dental injury, unless the teeth are dislodged, or if bleeding is noticed. However, on occasion children present with atypical injuries, or injuries which do not fit the trauma described by the accompanying adult. In these cases, the dentist must be alert to the possibility of non-accidental injury. Children who are being abused are in very severe and real danger. The dentist must be aware of this, as s/he has a responsibility to protect children, as do all adults. Thus, it is essential that the dentist takes a clear history, asking when and where the injury occurred and exactly what happened (so that s/he can compare the injury to the story and check that they are compatible). S/he must also find out who was at the scene at the time and the length of time between injury and presentation. Any inconsistencies in the history or disputes between the child and accompanying adult about how the injury occurred should be carefully noted. If the dentist is suspicious that all is not well, the child's GP should be contacted. The medical practice will then alert social services if they believe that there is a need. The doctor may ask you to refer the child for examination.

If your suspicion that abuse of a child has occurred is very strong, the police should be called. The child should not be left alone with the accompanying adult if it is they who are thought to be the perpetrator of the child's injuries.

On questioning Jess's mother, there was no obvious cause for the tooth's discoloration. There was also no sinus, nor did a periapical radiograph show any radiolucency, other than that associated with the crypt of the developing UL1.

Teeth which are darker than the other teeth in the arch are likely to be non-vital. Non-vitality may arise from trauma or from caries extending to the pulp. Often they are completely symptomless. Some will eventually cause an abscess and sinus at the apex (anterior deciduous and permanent teeth) or at the furcation (posterior deciduous teeth)

Unless there are signs of suppuration on either a radiograph (a radio-lucency) or in the mouth (sinus) the tooth can be monitored. If pus formation does occur, or if symptoms arise, then darkened teeth should be extracted.

In Jess's case, the dentist felt that the ULA was non-vital due to previous but unknown trauma and that it would therefore be better if it were removed so that the successor tooth would not be affected by any infection which might develop.

If a deciduous tooth is intruded by a blow, or if it is avulsed, damage to the underlying permanent successor tooth can occur. This is because the apex of the root of the deciduous tooth lies very close to the crypt of the developing permanent tooth.

However, injuries and blows to the deciduous teeth can cause two types of disruption to the formation of the permanent tooth. If the normal maturation of the enamel of the permanent tooth germ is interfered with, the permanent tooth may have a white or yellowish area of discoloration. Typically, in incisors, this will be on the buccal aspect of the crown. In more severe cases, the enamel tissue may be deficient.

This type of enamel disruption is thought to be caused by direct trauma from the deciduous tooth root, whilst in posterior teeth the enamel mal-formation is thought to be caused by chronic infection around the tooth. Teeth so affected are known as 'Turner teeth'.

If an intrusive injury to a deciduous incisor occurs at the stage when the permanent crown has calcified but the remainder of the tooth is still soft, the permanent tooth may become 'dilacerated'. That is, the tooth is 'bent' on its long axis. These teeth may erupt if the dilaceration is not severe but dilaceration must be considered if a permanent incisor is slow to come into the arch. Orthodontic traction can assist but very severely affected teeth will need to be extracted.

The dentist informed Jess's mother that the tooth was dead and needed to be removed.

The dentist is of the opinion that the tooth is non-vital because it is darker than the others, but there are no signs of infection. The dentist considered that there was a risk of infection developing and that such infection might affect the developing permanent UL1. The first question to consider is whether the dentist is correct in his diagnosis of non-vitality, and leading from that, whether there is a risk of damage, and what is the size of that risk, to the developing UL1.

The dentist has simply told the mother the tooth *needs* to be removed. If the risk of infection and damage is high, not quite a certainty but high, then the proposed extraction would seem to be the appropriate course of action. However, the dentist doesn't appear to have told the mother the reason or purpose for the extraction. It is essential for the purpose of enabling the mother to make an informed choice that the dentist does so. Even faced with the information of a high risk of damage it is still her choice to leave the tooth or extract it as advised. Whatever the risks of infection and of ensuing damage to the UL1 that is information that the mother needs in order to make an informed choice, perhaps involving Jess in the discussion, although she is a little young for her wishes to have much influence. The parent needs information to be able to balance risks against the cosmetic effect of premature loss of ULA for a couple of years and the likely effect of the extraction and any cosmetic blemishes to UL1.

Jess's mother agreed to the extraction and the dentist prepared to remove the tooth under local anaesthesia. At the point of extraction, Jess became very very distressed, almost hysterical. However, Jess's mother insisted that the dentist continue and helped to hold Jess still. The dentist managed to extract the tooth but Jess was inconsolable.

The General Dental Council (GDC) in 'Maintaining standards' suggests that the use of physical restraint is only justified in exceptional circumstances. The question here then is whether the circumstances described can be considered to be 'exceptional'. The GDC goes on to say that when faced with a child who is uncontrollable for whatever reason the dentist should consider ceasing treatment, making an appropriate explanation to the parent, and arranging future treatment rather than continuing.

Would such restraint be unlawful? Such a question is often answered by asking whether or not doing so was in the child's best interests. A better approach might be to ask whether or not it was clearly against the child's interests. If it is not against the child's interests and if there is valid parental consent it would appear to be a lawful course of action, provided it is not cruel or excessive

(S v McC [1972] AC 24). So we need to consider whether the mother's consent was a valid one and whether the actions taken were cruel or excessive. Finally, we need to determine whether the extraction could have been abandoned without harm.

Choosing to extract any symptomless tooth is a matter of weighing the costs and benefits of both treatment and of inaction. If the dentist does not do this *and* present his/her deliberations to the parent, the parent cannot be said to be being allowed to make an informed choice. In this instance, the costs and benefits are as follows:

- Removing the tooth ensures that Jess does not suffer the pain of an abscess. However, most non-vital deciduous incisors will develop a draining sinus without the child ever describing any symptoms. Unfortunately, there is not enough research data available to enable the dentist to express numerically the probability of these potential outcomes. S/he will only be able to assess the probability of the sequelae of action and inaction from his/her own experience, from what s/he was taught, and perhaps from audits undertaken in his/her practice.

- A further potential 'cost' of inaction would be the permanent successor being hypoplastic if infection arises. However, since the crown of the permanent central incisor is already largely formed at the age of 5, this risk is really only a theoretical one, and the enamel structure once formed will not be affected by the presence of suppuration.

Obviously, one of the issues a dentist and parent must consider when planning the extraction of a symptom-free deciduous tooth is whether doing so will affect the child's view of dentistry. It may be that the trauma of an extraction at an early age might be damaging to the child's future acceptance of dental care. If this happens, this one action might prejudice the child's ability to accept treatment for the remainder of their life. This is not necessarily very likely but should be considered, as all decisions should be taken with the child's best long-term as well as short term interests in mind.

After the extraction, the UL1 erupted a little earlier than normal but appeared normal, apart from some white flecks. The contralateral tooth UR1 was not similarly affected.

White flecks in enamel can have many causes. The most likely are either fluorosis or as a result of trauma to the deciduous dentition (see above).

Fluorosis would be diagnosed if the white flecks were generalized throughout the dentition, if the affected parts of the permanent dentition matched developmental stages, or if there were a history of potential over-exposure to fluoride ions (living in a fluoridated area plus, use of fluoride supplements, or a habit of toothpaste ingestion).

In contrast, trauma is more likely to be the cause of white patches of enamel if a single tooth is affected, if there is no history of (over) exposure to fluoride, or if parts of teeth from different stages of development are affected.

Sometimes, simple developmental defects occur which manifest as white marks in the enamel.

At the age of 8, Jess attended for her 6-monthly check-up as usual. (Her mother had continued to bring her after the extraction, and after three or four visits in which she was cajoled into an examination, Jess once again became cooperative.) Jess complained at this visit of having 'funny teeth'.

Deciduous teeth are much whiter than the permanent teeth and are smoother and smaller. Also, the deciduous dentition often occludes in an edge-to-edge way, which means that attrition is common, making the crown lengths even shorter.

Thus, when the permanent central incisors erupt, for the short period for which the deciduous laterals and canines are still present, the new central incisors tend to look abnormally large and rather yellow in comparison with their deciduous neighbours.

Also, the incisors will often erupt with a spacing and with a somewhat fan-like appearance. This is because the roots are crowded into a relatively small space, bounded by the unerupted crowns of the canines, whilst the teeth are erupting into a growing alveolus.

This is, somewhat unfortunately, often referred to as the 'ugly duckling' stage (around 8 years).

When the dentist enquired further, Jess said that her teeth were 'all yellowy' and that they were 'goofy'. On examination, Jess's teeth and occlusion were normal. The dentist told Jess's mother that there was no cause for concern with Jess's teeth and that she did not need treatment.

It took Jess some time to recover from the previous ordeal and this raises again the issue of whether the extraction was in Jess's best interests. Jess seems to have regained enough confidence and trust in the dentist to voice her own concerns in respect of the appearance of her teeth. The dentist should therefore be at great pains to discuss this with her after his examination. The dentist seems to have only discussed it with Jess's mother. There can be no doubt that at 8 years of age Jess is old enough to become involved in discussions about her teeth. How else will Jess learn to develop such skills and take an interest in her own health care? Surely, too, for relatively simple and, perhaps, unimportant matters her views should be taken into account. As one 8-year-old reported in a recent study of consent in dental care: 'I'd rather be involved because it's me they're doing it to.'

Jess's visits continued to be regular, and her oral hygiene perfect.

When Jess was about 12 years old, the dentist noticed that there was some gingival recession of the canine teeth.

Recession occurs on canines because:
- There may be a bony dehiscence on the buccal surface of the root.
- The canine is often more prominent in the line of the arch than other teeth so may receive more trauma from toothbrushing.

- It may be the area in the mouth that the patient first puts his/her tooth-brush freshly loaded with toothpaste, which is an abrasive.

Canines look darker because they have a larger bulk of dentine when compared with the other anterior teeth and this gives the appearance of yellowness.

If patients have recession they should be encouraged to modify their tooth-brushing technique. Most patients use a horizontal scrubbing motion which often fails to remove plaque from the gingival margins and interproximally. In patients with recession they should be encouraged to use a brush with softer bristles and to use a systematic approach so that all surfaces of the teeth are cleaned. The Bass technique in which the toothbrush bristles are placed at the gingival margin then rolled crownwards, is frequently advised.

When questioned, Jess explained that she did brush these teeth particularly carefully because, she said, they were very yellow. The dentist also noticed that the URE and ULE were showing no signs of exfoliation.

The dentist therefore took a periapical radiograph of each and discovered that UR5 and UL5 were missing.

Premolars are fairly commonly absent. Whilst missing teeth are normally con-genitally absent, occasionally premolar tooth germs are lost at the extraction of deciduous molar teeth. The second premolar tooth germ develops between the roots of the second deciduous molars. If these molar teeth require extraction before the roots have begun to resorb but after the premolar tooth germ has begun to develop, the tooth germ may be inadvertently removed during ex-traction. Whilst figures for such events are not available, such scenarios may account for at least some of the so-called 'congenitally absent' premolars. Clearly in Jess's case, however, the 5s are congenitally absent since no deciduous molars have been extracted.

If UL5 and UR5 are found to be missing, a decision needs to be made as to whether to extract the deciduous molars during the mixed dentition stage, in the hope that the space will close, or to maintain the URE and ULE.

If the latter decision is made, if the URE and ULE are lost in adult life then deci-sions must again be made as to whether to close the resultant spaces or to provide bridges (or even possibly implants or dentures) to produce an intact dentition.

The dentist advised Jess that she would have to look after her baby molar teeth very carefully, so that they would last. The dentist also made a brief note that Jess appeared to be rather under weight.

At the age of 14, Jess attended, looking extremely thin. She said that when she ate something cold, or even if very cold air got near to her teeth, they were painful. She also said that: her teeth were 'shrinking'. Her mother then said that she knew why Jess's teeth were getting shorter. She said she has read in the newspapers about soft drinks causing erosion. She asked the dentist to tell Jess to stop 'drinking all that rubbish'.

Bulimia is a recognized eating disorder characterized by frequent binge eating and enthusiastic dieting or severe restriction of food intake. Weight gain is controlled by self-induced vomiting and other behaviours including vigorous exercise and chronic use of laxatives and diuretics. Dentists do not treat the bulimia but the after-effects. The stomach acids from the induced vomiting bathing the teeth are responsible for the erosion of the enamel on the surfaces of teeth.

Bulimia is relatively common in adolescents and young adults. There is a trend for the condition to occur at younger ages. The majority of cases (9 in 10) are female. Approximately 1 to 4% of females between 18 and 30 years suffer from bulimia. A third of bulimics have a history of obesity. Similarly, a third suffered anorexia nervosa at some stage.

There are some classic features of bulimia apart from the dental signs. These include: callouses near the first knuckle of the index finger due to the knuckle grazing the incisors when the tip of the finger is stimulating the back of throat to encourage vomiting; rapid weight change of 5 to 20 lbs per week; frequent gum chewing (over six packs per day); excessive mouth wash use and/or suck-ing of mint sweets; brushing of teeth over seven times a day. Drinking of car-bonated drinks is also frequent and is the issue that Jess's mother has picked up on. Much of this use of highly flavoured agents is to disguise the tell-tale odour of having vomited and also to get rid of the unpleasant taste. The tissues of the mouth and surrounding skin and lips become dry from the nausea and the reduced salivary flow and parotid gland dysfunction. However, other more serious conditions can result, including dizziness, thirst, and fainting as a result of dehydration. Nail biting and ice chewing are common. Complaints of muscle cramps and general fatigue are characteristic. Blood vessels around the eyes are often broken due to the strain of repeated vomiting.

Diagnosis of bulimia should not be confused with related signs and symp-toms. Dry mouth can be caused by certain drugs such as antidepressants. Erosion can be caused by excessive grinding; however, the erosion of bulimic patients tends to feature on non-contact surfaces. Gum recession can be caused by rapid and enthusiastic toothbrusing. Discoloured teeth are common in regular tea or coffee drinkers. The sucking of citrus fruits, especially lemons, may also erode the tooth surfaces.

Suspected bulimic patients can be counselled to visit their general medical practitioner to seek assistance in what can become a debilitating condition which can put the sufferer at a marked health risk of heart attacks, de-hydration, constipation, alcohol and drug abuse, and depression. Approxi-mately 35 to 70% of bulimics are depressed. Stabilization of the patient's condition is important to allow dental treatment to continue.

There is evidence that patients suffering with eating disorders have sig-nificant errors of assessing their own body shape. Ingenious methods relying on sophisticated visual morphing software has shown that patients with an eating disorder overestimate their body image by an average of 28% and desired to be 25% thinner. Interestingly, satisfaction with the appearance of the teeth was not associated with the estimates of body image.

The mother's behaviour was noted by the dentist as being somewhat strange in the dental surgery setting. The mother was distressed at her daughter's continued use of carbonated drinks, as indicated by the mother saying the drinks are 'rubbish'. At 14 years of age there are likely to be disagreements between the parent and child. This would not be unusual in an adolescent–parent relationship. The child seeks greater independence and pushes at parentally determined boundaries of appropriate behaviour. The mother, however, was enlisting the dentist to exert a controlling influence on her child's behaviour. There is evidence in the literature that child psychopathology develops through poor childrearing practices. In respect to the development of child anxiety the parent is believed to become over-involved in the child's welfare to the point where the child learns to appreciate that they are vulnerable to various threats. The parent aims to prevent the child from experiencing stressful events in order to protect them. In Jess's case the mother appears to show some features of over-involvement. This is appreciated by the dentist (later on in the case description) as the parent is asked to leave the surgery while the dentist discusses with Jess some treatment options. Jess's mother appeared not to be overly protective during the extraction episode, although it could be argued that the parent wanted to prevent any lengthy further sessions of dental visiting to treat the infected tooth. Recent work does, however, support the view that mothers of anxious children do exhibit more intrusive involvement in their parenting style. Whether the parent causes their child to become anxious due to this over involvement or whether the anxious child triggers this parenting style when exhibiting anxiety-related behaviour is unclear at present. It is important, however, for dentists to recognize the parent who may be influencing the child patient unduly and preventing the child from developing independence and taking decisions about their own oral health. The taking of responsibility for their own health by the young person should be encouraged progressively during the teenage years.

Having listened to this rather strange history from Jess, the dentist tried to work out what was going on. On examination, he found that the incisal edges of Jess's teeth were thin and there was wear of the upper palatal surfaces. Also he could see wear facets on the cusps of the lower posterior teeth. The URE and ULE were completely smooth and at gingival level.

Erosion often occurs on the palatal surfaces of the upper anterior teeth and on the occlusal surfaces of the lower posterior teeth. It may also be seen on the labial surfaces of the upper anterior teeth, depending on the causative factor. The crowns may be shorter than normal, with thin enamel. The surfaces appear smooth and shiny. There may be loss of contour of the teeth with cupping of the incisal edges and molar/premolar cusps. Restorations may stand proud of the surrounding tooth tissue.

If soft drinks are the cause then tooth surface loss is usually seen on the palatal surfaces (and possibly the labial surfaces) of the upper incisors and the occlusal surfaces of the lower molars. In eating disorders the tooth surface loss may affect the palatal surfaces of the upper anterior and premolar teeth.

The dentist decided that Jess's diet did indeed have something to do with her worn teeth, but decided that the best option, in the first instance, was to recommend that Jess use a desensitizing toothpaste and come back in a month.

Dentine hypersensitivity can be managed in several ways. In most cases improvement can be obtained from using a sensitive formula toothpaste containing potassium nitrate. Sodium fluoride mouthwash used once daily for 1 month may also be used. If there is no relief with these options then a dentine bonding agent, resin-modified glass ionomer, or resin composite can be applied to the exposed areas of dentine.

If you have recognized erosion affecting a patient's teeth and are unsure of the cause then one approach is to tell the patient of all the possible, common causes. You might mention drinks, e.g. carbonated soft drinks, wine, beer; foodstuffs, e.g. citrus fruits; medications, e.g. vitamin C tablets; lifestyle factors, e.g. swimming; and medical conditions such as hiatus hernia, regurgitation, and eating disorders. The patient may recognize the cause and tell you or they may deny the possibility of any of the factors you have described. It is appropriate, however, to advise patients of the possible causes and they can then choose to take the advice on board, or not.

Jess's mother seemed unimpressed with this course of action but agreed to it, muttering about the 'rubbish Jess drank' as she left the surgery.

Health scares in the media are common. Research has shown that the media coverage is inversely proportional to the actual risk posed by an issue.

This is evident in Jess's case. Sugary drinks cause tooth decay and yet media coverage of this is relatively limited. Soft drinks can also cause erosion but the risk posed is actually less than that of caries. However, because of coverage in the media, Jess's mother is probably assuming that there is a direct causal effect between Jess's soft drink consumption and her painful, 'shrinking' teeth.

After a month, Jess returned, but said that her teeth were 'still shrinking' and that there had not been any improvement in the sensitivity. On examination, the teeth looked much the same as on the previous occasion but the dentist could not be sure. At this point, the dentist considered what options were available for Jess.

Resin composites would restore the appearance of the incisors and protect against sensitivity and further tooth surface loss. The resin composite would be applied directly to the worn palatal surfaces and short incisal edges, following use of a dentine bonding system. Jess is 14 years old and further growth and gingival retreat could be expected. This would make composites a good interim restorative option.

Palatal veneers in gold would protect against sensitivity and further tooth surface loss palatally but would not restore the incisal length. The gold would need to be sandblasted or heat-treated prior to luting with a chemically cured composite luting system.

Palatal veneers in composite or porcelain could be made and would have the advantage of improved appearance compared with gold. Porcelain may be more liable to fracture depending on the occlusion. If the veneers were lipped over the incisal edges they would increase the incisal length. A join may be visible on the labial tooth surface between the tooth and the veneer.

Labial veneers if placed would require replacing in the future as one would expect further gingival retreat in a 14-year-old and this would result in possibly unsightly veneer margins being visible.

Crowns are not really appropriate at this age if they can be avoided.

A treatment plan was drawn up in discussion with Jess (but not her mother who the dentist excluded from the discussion). When it was explained that food could affect her teeth, Jess agreed to see a dietician about her eating habits.

Jess's mother was very against Jess seeing anyone else about what she ate.

When she was 18, Jess went to the surgery to tell the dentist that she hated the appearance of the URE and ULE. These were worn down and discoloured, and Jess felt they were visible when she smiled. The dentist thought Jess looked well, although still slightly under weight.

The retained teeth could be simply left *in situ* but Jess should be advised that the teeth would be unlikely to survive beyond around the age of 40 years. Alternatively, the URE and ULE could be extracted. Orthodontic treatment would then be required in order to close the spaces.

The teeth could also be extracted and implants placed to restore spaces. Alternatively, the appearance of URE and ULE could be improved with either direct composite restorations or composite crowns but this would not offer Jess a permanent solution regarding URE and ULE.

The URE and ULE were extracted and the spaces closed orthodontically. Jess then went to university. She had achieved extremely high grades at 'A' level and was going to study medicine. The dentist wondered whether he should alert the university authorities to Jess's eating disorder.

The dentist wondered whether or not he ought to alert the university authorities to the eating disorder which he thinks Jess has. It does not appear that Jess has told the dentist that she has an eating disorder. An eating disorder is the dentist's own diagnosis based on dental changes. Jess has not confided in him but that does not mean that the dentist's suspicion of an eating disorder is not confidential information. If true, and Jess does indeed have an eating disorder, contacting Jess's intended university would, without any doubt, be a breach of confidentiality.

The principle of confidentiality in health care arises from the relationship of trust between the health-care provider and the patient. Without that trust and the assurance of confidentiality two differing consequences may result. First, a patient may not divulge information about themselves which is relevant to their required care because they do not wish others to know about it. Such concealment could be detrimental to their health. A second, and probably worse scenario, is that patients may fail to seek treatment or help for their illnesses and problems because they do not wish the world at large to know about those illnesses or problems. For those reasons confidentiality in health care remains of paramount importance.

As a general, and very broad principle, breach of confidentiality can be justified when the public interest (not what the public is interested in) outweighs the individual's private interests, or when the law demands. It can, however, be argued that, ethically, demands of the law do not always justify a breach of confidentiality.

Therefore, we need to determine what might justify the dentist informing Jess's university? What is the dentist's purpose in doing so? What perceived benefit will be gained? It seems that the dentist has not even discussed his concerns with Jess's doctor. Such a discussion with a patient's GP would probably be accepted by most as not being a breach of confidentiality, unless it had been expressly proscribed by Jess.

So the dentist's decision must rest on whether there is any possible public interest in the university being informed about Jess's suspected eating disorder and, if so, whether that interest outweighs Jess's private interests.

Aged 24, Jess returned to the surgery saying that she was getting married in 3 months' time and that she definitely wanted her teeth made whiter and longer. On questioning she stated that she had not been able to complete her medical degree, after having had a year off after studying medicine for 2 years. She had decided that she may have chosen to do the medical degree for the wrong reasons, related more to the wishes of her parents rather than following her real interests.

Jess could have lateral and palatal veneers placed. The palatal veneers could be in gold, providing good wear characteristics and ease of adjustment, or in porcelain, giving good aesthetics. Porcelain labial veneers would offer better long-term aesthetics than composite veneers. The double veneer technique prevents the loss of the contact areas that occurs when crowns are provided.

An alternative treatment would be resin-bonded crowns and these are often used for erosion cases. They require minimal preparation and are full-coverage all-ceramic restorations that are bonded to the tooth using a resin composite luting system.

A final possibility would be metal ceramic crowns but these would require much tooth destruction and are therefore not an appropriate option for a 24-year-old with erosion of her upper anterior teeth.

In a dentist's career the possibility of treating a patient with an extreme pre-occupation with the appearance of the teeth is moderate as the incidence of a mental condition known as dysmorphophobia is rare. However, when encountered the dentist is recommended to seek assistance from other members of the primary or secondary health services, such as a psychiatrist or clinical psychologist. The condition has been renamed in the modern diagnostic systems as body dysmorphic disorder (BDD). It is defined as a preoccupation with an imagined or minor defect in appearance. Two sets of symptoms are recognizable. First, there is excessive concern with an imagined defect, and secondly, there is evidence of clinically significant distress or functional impairment. Other mental dysfunction cannot be implicated. The key to identifying whether a patient has the features of this condition is the degree to which his or her concern affects their normal routine of work or relationships with family and friends. A patient who is unable to communicate at an interpersonal level because of his/her fixation on the appearance of a feature of his/her physique would be worth referring for a psychiatric or detailed psychological assessment. Clues to patients that may be dysmorphophobic include:

- An inability to dismiss negative thoughts about the physical feature, so that the difficulties expressed by the patient take on a clear obsessional quality.
- Continual and frequent requests for improvements to the shape, colour, and position of the object of preoccupation (e.g. tooth or teeth).
- An inability to consider that a request should be delayed to consider other possible options.
- High levels of distress displayed (anger, tearfulness, agitation, threats of abuse to staff) when suggestion is made to the patient that there is no suitable treatment available or required.
- Appeals to the staff of the practice that not providing treatment would have dire consequences, such as an inability to return to work or enter or maintain a close confiding relationship.
- A distinctly distorted view of the appearance of the object in question. For example, a preoccupation about the shade of tooth colour when from objective assessment the shade is close to normative values for the age of the individual.
- History of previous mental health difficulties or drug or alcohol abuse.

In Jess's case the level of distress, although relatively marked, does not appear to have reached clinical levels requiring professional help. There is evidence, however, that she has a strong interest in the appearance of her teeth. This may be a reflection of her past behaviour, which showed definite evidence for chronic and frequent consumption of carbonated drinks. It is speculative, but possible, that Jess may feel somewhat to blame for the condition of her teeth. It may therefore be expected that she should focus on their appearance. Evidence for undue preoccupation is not strong. She has entered into a commitment to get married and has a wedding planned in a few months. The request for attempting to improve her appearance for the wedding day may not be unreasonable from a psychological viewpoint. Had she broached this request with an ultimatum that without the improvements to her appearance she would call the event off, then this should trigger the concern of the dentist to consider her mental health.

BIBLIOGRAPHY

Bartlett D. Bleaching discoloured teeth. *Dental Update* 2001; **28**(1): 14–18.

Fain MP. Recognition and management of eating disorders in the dental office. *Dental Clinics of North America* 2003; **47**(2): 395–410.

Feinmann C. *The Mouth, the Face and the Mind*. Oxford University Press: Oxford, 1999.

General Dental Council. *Maintaining Standards*. www.gdc-uk.org/pdfs/ms_full_nov2001.pdf

Hudson JL, Rapee RM. Parent–child interactions and anxiety disorders: an observational study. *Behavior Research and Therapy* 2001; **39**(12): 1411–1427.

Ibbetson R, Eder A. *Tooth Surface Loss*. BDJ Books: London, 2000.

King J. Dental care for children. In: Lambden P (ed.) *Dental Law and Ethics*, pp. 49–63. Radcliffe Medical Press: Oxford, 2002.

King J, Hillier S, Duyal L. *Consent in Dental Care*. King's Fund: London, 2000.

Milosevic A, Thomas J, Mitzman S. Satisfaction with dento-facial appearance in the eating disorders. *European Journal of Prosthodontics and Restorative Dentistry* 2003; **11**(3): 125–128.

O'Brien M. Children's dental health in the United Kingdom in 1993. Reports office of Population Censuses and Survey. Social Surveys Division: London, 1994.

Shearer AC, Mellor AC. *Treatment Planning in Primary Dental Care*. Oxford University Press: Oxford, 2003.

Todd J, Dodd J. Children's dental health in the United Kingdom in 1983. Great Britain Office of Population Censuses and Surveys. Social Surveys Division: London, 1985.

Index

erosion of upper 140
fractured 113
immature 115, 118
palatal view of erosion 140
upper, restored with resin bonded crowns
  141
infection 132
focal 7
peri-implant 132
universal precautions against 53–4
informed choice 93, 138, 144, 145
informed consent 93, 103
inhalation sedation 85, 104–5, 124, 125
injections 113
inferior dental block 82
injury
significant 54
traumatic 142–3
International Association for the Study of
  Pain 94
interviewing, motivational 70
irreversible pulpitis 128

Japan 41

ketoacidosis 23

law of contract 98
learned helplessness 45–6, 48
Ledermix 51
legal issues 82
lidocaine 98
lip lacerations 124
litigation 61, 75
loading 132
local anaesthesia 72, 73, 83, 98, 125–6
locus of control 80, 88–9, 100, 103, 105
locus of responsibility 80

'Maintaining standards' 18, 127, 144
malocclusions 13, 111–12, 115, 117,
  118, 135

mandibular fracture 121
medical history 37, 52
medication 5, 18–19
methadone 51–2
  programme 36–7
Modified Dental Anxiety Scale 8, 101
molars
first permanent 47
lower 82
permanent 34
monoamine oxidase inhibitors 19
moral obligation 122
motivational interviewing 70
mouthguards 61, 69–70, 117, 134
mutualistic relationship 90

National Health Service 75
Regulations 16
Smoker's Helpline 87
nitrous oxide 104
non-maleficence 50, 91
non-vitality 81, 143, 144, 145
note keeping 114, 119, 124, 127

occlusally carious teeth 3
occlusion, poor 13
opioid drugs 52
oral functioning 85–6
Oral Health Impact Profile 106
Oral Health-Quality of Life UK 106
oral hygiene, poor 35
oral sepsis 7
outcomes, poor 62
overdenture 4, 5
overgrowth, gingival 4, 19

pain 82–3, 94–8, 102, 115, 128, 129
palatal veneers 151
parental responsibility 122
paternalistic relationship 90
perceived efficacy 70
peri-implant infections 132
periodontal disease 23–4
periradicular
periodontitis 81
radiolucency 63
surgery 63, 68